W

Effective

Second Edition

Effective People

LEADERSHIP AND ORGANISATION DEVELOPMENT IN HEALTHCARE

Second Edition

STEPHEN PROSSER

Professor of Leadership and Organisation Development
University of Glamorgan
and Founding Chief Executive
NHS Staff College Wales

JET LIBRARY

Radcliffe Publishing
Oxford • New York

Radcliffe Publishing Ltd
18 Marcham Road
Abingdon
Oxon OX14 1AA
United Kingdom

www.radcliffe-oxford.com
Electronic catalogue and worldwide online ordering facility

British Library Cataloguing in Publication Data
A catalogue record for this book is available from the British Library.

ISBN-13: 978 184619 391 0

The paper used for the text pages of this book
is FSC certified. FSC (The Forest Stewardship
Council) is an international network to promote
responsible management of the world's forests.

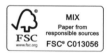

Typeset by Pindar NZ, Auckland, New Zealand
Printed and bound by TJI Digital, Padstow, Cornwall, UK

For Thomas, Daniel and Simon –
the three best sons a man could have

Contents

Preface to the second edition

When I wrote the preface to the first edition of this book, I wanted to convince potential and actual readers that they would find in its pages helpful material written by someone with experience of working in healthcare and manufacturing as well as with senior civil servants – and by an academic familiar with the key literature. I set out to show a combination of practice, theory and policy that could be applied in practice.

That still holds true, but as a result of my experiences since 2005 (and before, but unmentioned in the first edition) I also wanted to produce this version with my experiences as a patient firmly in mind. In 2000 and again in 2006, if it had not been for the skills of clinicians and others, I would have died – and I owe them a debt I shall never be able to repay. Therefore, I have also reviewed and partly re-written this book from the perspective of a patient, in addition to looking at the material through managerial, academic and policy lenses. This does not mean that I have changed my mind about what I wrote earlier, but it has become more important to me because I believe with a passion that we need effective people working in effective organisations for the benefit of the patients they serve.

In these pages you will find a rich mixture of the best in leadership and organisation development practice and theory, based on a lifetime of studying and applying the principles of why some healthcare and other organisations and individuals succeed and why some fail.

For the best part of 30 years I worked as a senior executive in the public sector. In 1995, I became the founding chief executive of the NHS Staff College Wales, and oversaw its spectacular tenfold growth, and before that I worked for many years in a number of strategic NHS posts. As an internal healthcare consultant I have worked closely with chief executives and their boards (and also with senior people in other public sector organisations), with a range of levels of civil servants (including permanent secretaries) and with university senior managers up to vice-chancellor level. I was also a senior manager in the nationalised manufacturing sector with British Steel. Thus I have experience of life at the top of a variety of public-sector organisations, and my academic interests have come to the fore in more recent years as a professor in a university business school.

Throughout those 35 years I made sure that I brought together theory and practice. I believe that the best in management theory can help healthcare organisations and individuals to prosper, and similarly I believe that it is essential for management experience to inform the development of applied research. This combination of practice and theory has also helped me to work with senior civil servants as they tackled issues concerned with policy development, and in return I have ensured that my knowledge of the operation of Government is fed back into my work with clinicians, healthcare managers and academics.

Therefore I have first-hand experience of three components of the public sector, namely within healthcare, as someone who has worked closely with civil servants and understands how they deal with Government policy, and as an academic who knows the leadership and organisation development literature thoroughly. Far more importantly, I understand the cultural differences between each of these three components, and I spend a large amount of my time bringing together my knowledge of policy development and implementation, my first-hand appreciation of the challenges of running a healthcare organisation and my in-depth understanding of leading-edge practice. The three come together to help to make healthcare, and the rest of the public sector, more effective.

There you have it – these are my credentials for writing this book. It is a book about the best in management practice and academic theory, flavoured with an appreciation of the world of the Government policy maker, and sprinkled with large doses of practical, down-to-earth common sense taken from my internal consultancy experience with healthcare clients, together with my own leadership and management adventures as an NHS chief executive.

At first I proposed to call this book *Misunderstanding Organisations*, an intended play on the title of Charles Handy's classic work *Understanding Organizations*.[1] His masterpiece, which has now gone through several editions, has sold hundreds of thousands – perhaps millions – of copies around the world. Its success and popularity are thoroughly deserved – it is a superb textbook on the theory of organisations and management, and Handy has a rightly merited position in the pantheon of great business writers.

The reason for originally choosing the title *Misunderstanding Organisations* was to emphasise a sub-text of this book. I wanted to ask some healthcare organisations and their leaders the following fundamental question. If we know so much about the way healthcare organisations should be run and how people should be led, as a result of a welter of academic and practical experience, then why is it that many organisations and their leaders get many things wrong? In other words, why are there so many *misunderstanding organisations*, organisations that misunderstand?

They know how change should be managed effectively, but they rarely achieve this. They know the essentials of leadership and how it differs from and yet complements management, but they do not necessarily practise it. They understand the importance of developing the full potential of their people, but this is usually relegated to next year's list of top priorities. If you ask them how their healthcare organisation is performing in these areas, they will reply with an eloquence that belies the reality of their position. So an important sub-text of this book focuses on those healthcare organisations that understand how they should act, yet manage to misunderstand and to get things wrong. However, the more I thought about the title of the book, the more concerned I became that to call it *Misunderstanding Organisations* was to invite misunderstanding in and of itself. People might even think that the title should be interpreted in some perverse way as an attempt by me to present a book that sets out to give a false picture of organisations – how to misunderstand organisations!

So I decided that the book should be called *Effective People: leadership and organisation development in healthcare* – a far more conventional title and one that avoids the potential for confusion and even further misunderstanding. However, the sub-text of the book remains, although I have deliberately avoided the practice of littering the book with repeated references such as '. . . and that is yet another example of where healthcare organisations misunderstand'. To write in such a style would be inelegant, unnecessary and would run the risk of annoying the reader.

The main message of the book concerns the effectiveness of people – although there are times when this is best demonstrated by highlighting ineffective behaviour – and the leadership and development of the healthcare organisations in which they reside. The book sets out the *disciplines and attitudes for effective people and their organisations* and, in a range of chapters, examines key attitudes and disciplines that will result in positive gain. Some of the chapters are quite long and others are shorter. Some use metaphors to demonstrate the main learning points and some use anecdotes (all perfectly legitimate techniques for unravelling the mystery of running an organisation in my opinion). Other chapters are essay-like, as they explore an issue, while some may appear to be more akin to a healthcare management checklist. Whatever the approach used within it, each chapter will challenge the reader to examine how they function in their organisation.

An added benefit of the layout of the book is that the reader is able to dip into the book's chapters in any order – whichever one happens to catch the eye first, or the one that best meets the time available, or the one that addresses the most important issue confronting the reader at present.

This book will set the reader thinking. It asks them to look at people and healthcare organisational issues from different perspectives. It sets out to challenge the reader about the things that take place every day of their working life. It asks them to think about those activities objectively and in a way that is determined only by the criterion of effectiveness. The fundamental question is 'Do your actions have a positive effect on the people you lead and on the overall performance of your healthcare organisation?' The reader will not need persuading that there are actually some managers and leaders whose actions do in fact have a detrimental impact on their staff and organisation. You almost certainly do not belong to that category of person – you are the type of person who realises that there are people who want to be led by you, and this book will challenge you to respond positively and effectively.

I love books – the look of them, the feel of them and even the smell of them. Above all, I love the fact that even if they contain just one new idea, that is enough to inspire me to tackle a new challenge or to rethink the way in which I am approaching some aspect of my job. I am also aware that books can be objects that merely gather dust on my shelves, and that there is a danger of believing that I am a master of all the untried techniques outlined on their pages. In that way books can be deceptive. My hope is that you will use this book frequently, that you will see its pages as a challenge, and that the deliberate changes of writing style in the book will increase the value of the book for you. Above all, my hope is that you, the people who work with you, and your area of healthcare will prosper, and if this book has played even a small part in that I shall be an extremely happy man.

Stephen Prosser
Llandeilo
Carmarthenshire
October 2009

REFERENCE

1 Handy C (1999) *Understanding Organizations*. Penguin, Harmondsworth.

About the author

Stephen Prosser (PhD) is a university professor, public-sector consultant and former NHS chief executive. In October 2001, he became Professor of Leadership and Organisation Development at the University of Glamorgan, where he contributes to doctoral and masters programmes, serves as the Business School's ethics champion, and is a member of several academic committees. He undertakes consultancy work across the public sector, working with senior civil servants to permanent secretary level, with public sector chief executives and their boards, and with university vice-chancellors. He was the founding chief executive of the NHS Staff College Wales in 1995, and led its substantial six-year growth and achievements in leadership development and consequential service improvement. He is the author of four books and monographs on leadership and public policy, including key health service issues, and is a regular conference speaker. His doctoral work concerned organisational learning in the public sector. In 2003, he became one of the first Companions of the Institute of Healthcare Management, in recognition of his contribution to professional development in the NHS. He is also a fellow of the Chartered Institute of Personnel and Development, the Chartered Management Institute and the Royal Society for Arts. He is a trustee of a national charity and sits on the editorial advisory board of the *International Journal of Servant-Leadership*.

Acknowledgements

As I set out on a postgraduate course almost 30 years ago, my wife Lesley gave me a card to wish me every success. The card had a phenomenal effect on me, and to this day I have it on a shelf in my office. The front cover shows a child's embroidery, and it contains the most appropriate words imaginable:

> How truly blest are they who
> Leisure find – to improve the little
> Garden of the mind – that grateful
> Tillage best rewards our pains –
> Sweet is the labour certain are our
> Gains – the rising Harvest never
> Mocks our toil – Secure of fruit
> If we manure the soil.

Even after 30 years the card is still a cherished possession, and although it is beginning to fade, I can just make out that the embroidery was the work of Christian Ann Nevitt, aged 11 years, who produced it in 1801.

Many a time Lesley and I would laugh about the importance of 'manuring the soil' but my gratitude to her extends far beyond a mere card. Her commitment to learning has been a true inspiration, and I have learned more from her than anyone would imagine.

I have also been extremely fortunate to work with a wide range of people, in healthcare and elsewhere, who taught me valuable lessons and who were an inspiration. There were managers and leaders – some of the cerebral variety, others who taught me the tactics of being 'streetwise', and some who gave me a hard time, sometimes quite unfairly and sometimes fairly, but who taught me important principles about the leadership of people. There have also been senior civil servants whose approach to issues of policy and operations was a revelation and a source of much helpful learning.

Over the years, both as a senior health service manager and as an academic, I have been inspired by many writers, particularly Richard Beckhard, Rosabeth Moss Kanter and Peter Senge. You can imagine, therefore, the enormous benefit I received from 'sitting at their feet' on various occasions when they presented invitational master classes in London. Above all, I wish to acknowledge my gratitude to the writings of Robert K. Greenleaf – his contribution has been inspirational. Their writing and teaching have helped my thinking and formed my approach to leadership, organisation development and management, and their insights into the world of work can hardly be bettered.

Then there are the UK academics. During my time at Warwick Business School I had the privilege of being taught by people of the calibre of Professor (now Sir) George Bain and Professor Keith Sisson.

Finally, a big 'thank you' to the team at Radcliffe Publishing Ltd for making this book possible, and especially to Gillian Nineham for her guidance and encouragement.

Disciplines

CHAPTER 1

Leadership

In today's dynamic world, the business environment is constantly changing. It is driven by the economic situation – both global and domestic advances in technology, changing markets, regulatory change and fierce competition. Never has leadership – and continuity of leadership – been more important.[1]

This is some claim from George Cox, recent Director General of the UK's Institute of Directors, and he is not alone. Acclaimed leadership writers, Rob Goffee and Gareth Jones, writing in the wake of the 2009 financial crisis believe:

As we struggle through the most serious economic crisis since 1929, it's clear that we do not yet know what the business landscape will look like when we do finally emerge from the recession. What we do know, however, is that leadership is more important than ever and organisations that are well led have much more chance of surviving these turbulent times.[2]

Recognition of the existence and importance of leadership has been around since the dawn of time: the Old Testament discussed it, as did the Icelandic sagas and the Greek and Latin classics. Confucius and Plato were interested in leadership, and the *Odyssey* even advised leaders on maintaining their social distance: 'The leader, mingling with the vulgar host, is in the common mass of matter lost'.[3] Despite this longevity in the practice of leadership, Cox, Goffee and Jones may well be right. Leadership may never have been so important, and in recent times the prominence given to it, in an ever-burgeoning and unprecedented literature, seems to support this claim. Organisations realise that effective leadership will provide them with a competitive edge over rivals and help to continue the transformation of their organisations.

In healthcare, there is widespread recognition of the importance of leadership for the provision of effective services. The website of Donald Berwick's influential Institute of Healthcare Improvement (www.ihi.org/ihi) is replete with examples of the impact of leadership on effective patient care, not least as evidenced through work on patient safety including the prevention of avoidable deaths. In England, the health services chief executive has established and will chair a potentially powerful National Leadership Council on the premise that:

> Leadership is the vital ingredient that can make all the difference to the quality
> of care that our patients experience. Great leadership, which focuses on improv-
> ing services for patients, will help transform the NHS.[4]

Whether there is evidence of a link between leadership development and positive patient experiences will be considered later in this chapter.

The UK Government saw leadership and management as such an important
issue that in 2000 the then Secretaries of State for Education and Employment
and for Trade and Industry established the Council for Excellence in Management
and Leadership, the aim being 'to develop a strategy to ensure that the UK has
the managers and leaders of the future to match the best in the world'. The
Council took to its task with relish and set out a compelling vision statement
(the realism of which will be judged soon) to underpin its recommendations:

> By 2010, the UK will be seen as a world leader in developing and deploying
> management and leadership capability for the twenty-first century.

Across many sectors of the economy major international companies continue
to invest in the development of their existing and future leadership talent, as
evidenced in books such as Fuller and Goldsmith's *The Leadership Investment –
How The World's Best Organizations Gain Strategic Advantage Through Leadership
Development*.[5] Although the widespread interest in leadership is commendable,
there is a danger that certain managers will see leadership – or possibly have
already seen it – as the latest panacea for all of their problems. Where that happens, leadership is in danger of becoming merely the latest fad. These managers
will be tempted to believe that 'If only we had the right type of leadership in this
organisation most of our problems would be solved and most of our challenges
would be met', and they say it with the same simpering optimism that greeted
the last managerial panacea they discovered.

This growing interest in leadership is reflected in the ever-increasing number
of books published on the subject (and the books, no doubt, are feeding the
frenzied interest in leadership), and the volume of reports from Government
departments and professional bodies examining and recommending the need for
more leadership to drive forward the public and private sectors. I am more than
willing to declare my belief that effective leadership is critically important in all
organisations, whatever sector they may occupy. However, I am also concerned
(for reasons I shall elaborate upon in other chapters) when I see the subject of
leadership being treated superficially and as the latest 'quick fix' to solve an array
of organisational or specific healthcare needs. As I write these words (in 2009)
I have on my desk a brochure from a well-known UK health-related institution
inviting me to attend a conference session where I will be able to learn how
to: adapt my leadership style to drive large-scale change; develop a commercial
culture of innovation and transformation; and ensure change has positive outcomes for both staff and patients. Some claims for a session programmed to run
from 10.10 to 10.40! There is rarely such a thing as a quick fix in an organisation
and for leadership to take its proper place and help the organisation to prosper,
leadership must be understood properly and practised effectively.

Andrew Pettigrew, the distinguished academic and analyst, provided balance with regard to the place of leadership within an organisation in an article entitled 'Does leadership make a difference to organisational performance?' Pettigrew contended:

> . . . although leaders are important and leader effects are quite crucial, we shouldn't concentrate our attentions on leaders alone. Indeed, my belief about the links between innovation, change and performance is that we should think about fixing the system, and not just the people. This is not to rule out the significance of people, but it does mean looking at a wider set of factors in assessing why things do change and why performance goes up and down . . . easy assumptions about leadership effects should be avoided, especially given the tendency to over-attribute them. But you can't make the contrary conclusion – to say that leaders have no effect. The problem is to balance out the competing explanations.[6]

WHAT IS LEADERSHIP?

> I can't tell you what it is, but I know it when I see it.
>
> Supreme Court Justice's much publicised (and possibly
> apocryphal) comment about pornography

Leadership is a complex subject, yet its complexity does not prevent many people from wanting to reduce the whole subject to a user-friendly definition of no more than six or seven words. They want a simple, easy-to-remember, slogan-type definition that will sum up the subject in as few memorable words as possible.

Leadership cannot be understood by such simplistic methods. It is necessary first of all to understand many different perspectives on the subject, and secondly, to comprehend the many complementary activities that impact upon its practice. I like very much Keith Grint's[7] demonstration of this complexity in his description of four quite different ways of understanding leadership:

➤ **Person**: is it WHO 'leaders' are that makes them leaders?
➤ **Result**: is it WHAT 'leaders' achieve that makes them leaders?
➤ **Position**: is it WHERE 'leaders' operate that makes them leaders?
➤ **Process**: is it HOW 'leaders' get things done that makes them leaders?

It is only when someone has examined leadership comprehensively that they can begin to declare an understanding, and even then they may feel that their studies have merely skimmed the surface. However, I would not want to carry the point of leadership complexity as far as leadership guru Warren Bennis in his description of the depth of leadership studies:[8]

> So there are two kinds of subjects that we academics tackle. Some, like fly-fishing or English seventeenth-century poetry, can be plumbed to their depths. Others, like leadership, are so vast and complex that they can only be explored.

Even if he has a point (although my English-language colleagues would dispute his reference to plumbing the depths of seventeenth-century poetry), the best application of his quote is to demonstrate to those who wish to reduce the subject of leadership to six or seven words that it cannot be explained in such a manner. I find that to develop a proper understanding of leadership it is necessary, in the first place, to start with the *negatives* and to describe in clear terms what leadership is not. Only then is it possible to move on to a *positive* description of leadership. Experience with vast numbers of healthcare managers and clinicians has taught me that there are typically five common misunderstandings about the subject of leadership. These are what can be called the *'five negatives'* of leadership.

The five negatives of leadership

1 *It is possible to provide a 'bumper-sticker' or 'fridge-magnet' explanation of leadership.* This attempt to explain leadership usually starts with the words 'Leadership is . . .' and ends with some simplistic explanation that, quite frankly, leaves more questions unanswered than answered. There is no glib answer to the question 'What is leadership?', even though there is continual pressure on leadership experts to sum up their entire field of enquiry in a few well-chosen words. I have lost count of the number of times I have been asked this question. The most recent occasion was at an international healthcare conference and when I explained to the enquirer that a short answer was impossible he respected my position and understood that short simple questions do not always have short simple answers. Instead, we decided to have another glass of wine and discuss some other imponderables of life.

2 *Leaders are only to be found at the top of the organisation.* This is the second common misunderstanding. It is what I call the 'Churchill and Mandela syndrome', where people believe that someone can only be a leader if they demonstrate qualities akin to those of great men such as Churchill and Mandela and occupy a place near the top of their hospital chain of command. The error lies in the belief that leadership can only come from the top of the organisation, and a failure to recognise that leadership is practised at all levels in the organisation, from the hospital ward or the GP's surgery to the oak-panelled boardroom. To think otherwise is to miss the leadership contribution made daily by a large percentage of nurses, doctors, porters and others in the organisation, in small acts that are often not classified as leadership, but which their colleagues recognise as indispensable. To confine leadership to the rarefied stratosphere of the senior people in the organisation is not a surprising error when one realises that the early studies of leadership, conducted between the 1930s and 1950s, did just that. They concerned themselves with the *great man* or *trait approach* and tried to identify the distinguishing qualities or characteristics that exemplified great leaders. The studies showed that there was no single set of such characteristics or traits, but the preoccupation with studying the great men – and, latterly and rightly, great women – has lasted and is still reflected in books being published today.

3 *'Tell me what I need to do to be a great leader!* This is a very tempting invitation!

However, it is almost impossible to do this without an in-depth understanding of the individual who is making the request and of the part of the health service in which they work . . . The nature of effective leadership depends on a variety of factors, and although it is possible to give a set of general pointers, genuine and helpful advice can only be given after there has been a period of diagnosis. I will say more about this later.

4 *Leaders are born, not made.* Ask any parent or schoolteacher and they will be able to provide evidence to substantiate a claim that leaders are born, not made. Leadership qualities can be seen in children at an early age, and many children seem to have a natural inclination – a gene – that makes them able and willing to lead others. Sometimes it appears as an ability to 'boss others around', which is often not the most attractive of qualities, but unquestionably there is something that sets some children apart as leaders from an early age. However, conceding that there is a genetic aspect to leadership is not the same thing as taking the view that because some people are born with a natural ability to lead, other people are doomed to be followers all their lives. Genetically inclined 'followers' can learn leadership skills and become effective leaders themselves. The analogy I use to make this point is taken from the world of tennis. I know that no matter how much I worked at it I would never have become another Pete Sampras or Roger Federer – I just did not have the natural athletic ability that top sportsmen need. However, I also know that if I had practised my tennis every day and been coached by a real expert, my serve and backhand would be very much better than they are at present. Training would have had a major impact on my tennis ability. It is exactly the same with leadership. You might never become the Federer of the leadership world, but your leadership performance can be enhanced dramatically.

As someone who has used that tennis example as a metaphor for leadership for many years, you can imagine my pleasure when I read about a revolutionary tennis coaching system in *The Sunday Times*:[9]

> According to Brad Langevad, a biomechanics expert and former professional tennis player, the way most people play tennis is fundamentally incorrect. To prove it, he has developed a scientific system which he claims can improve a player's technique in less than an hour.

Professional and amateur players are queuing up to benefit from his training sessions. It appears that:

> Langevad's system is the result of 12 years' scientific research into maximising performance and minimising sports injury. He became fascinated with how the human body moves when striking a ball, and began to wonder whether the perfect shot existed and, if so, who had it . . . he discovered that despite a few flawed idiosyncrasies there is an ideal body movement that produces the most effective serve, forehand, backhand and smash.

My analogy is complete. You might not become the Federer or Sampras of leadership, but with the right development you can become a far better leader than you are at present, and an excellent one when judged against most standards for leadership. Before leaving this point I must record the amusing insight given by John Maxwell.[10] He says there are three origins of leadership: nature, nurture and never. Surely, experience teaches us that some have a natural talent, others can develop it and some are just hopeless cases.

5 *Leaders come in one shape and size.* This is the final misunderstanding. Although people will rarely say that leaders only come in one shape and size, it is often this belief that forms their understanding of leadership, and the belief surfaces when they discuss their views on leadership. The belief has often been formed, quite subconsciously, by looking at the type of leaders that are successful in their part of the health system and concluding that they represent the model or ideal for leadership. There are still many healthcare chief executives who impersonate Frank Sinatra by convincing their people that to be successful as leaders they must do it 'My Way'. This results in people deifying one style of leadership that has been successful for them, but the chief executive, unwisely and possibly manipulatively, is expecting all of the followers to emulate his or her accomplishments and to copy his or her style of being a leader. This is a dangerous practice, and where it exists it inevitably leads to serious problems in the longer term for the organisation. It is important to appreciate that leadership comes in all shapes and sizes, and that this diversity or richness of approaches is an actual benefit to the world of healthcare. Diversity is to be welcomed and celebrated, and healthcare organisations that follow a single model of leadership would do well to set out to encourage a more diverse approach among their leaders.

SO 'WHAT IS LEADERSHIP?'

If these are the five popular misconceptions about leadership, then it behoves me to set out what I consider to be the proper definition of leadership – to move from the *negative* to the *positive*. At the end of the day it is impossible to refuse a request for information from a manager or clinician and to sit in an academic ivory tower protesting that an answer could not possibly be forthcoming in anything less than a three-hour tutorial. There is a need for people like me to be able to answer a request for clarification and to say something about the depths of leadership in a style that can be communicated in few words. I acknowledge immediately that this is a difficult task and invite others to criticise the approach I am taking. My approach is based on experience of working with various leaders, and when I am encouraged to produce my own set of leadership 'bumper stickers', these are the ones that I have found to resonate with clinicians and managers, and with other leaders across the public service. My contention is as follows.

1 Leadership is demonstrated through a set of qualities, attributes or characteristics

Most of the highly regarded leadership books will set out what they consider to be the characteristics of effective leaders. Richard Daft,[11] drawing on the work of

Bass and Stogdill, lists personal characteristics under the sub-headings of physical characteristics, intelligence and ability, personality, social characteristics, work-related characteristics, and social background. Daniel Goleman, *et al.*[12] reveal their *Leadership Styles in a Nutshell* to be visionary, coaching, affiliative, democratic, pacesetting and commanding. Kouzes and Posner,[13] within their definition of leadership as 'the art of mobilising others to want to struggle for shared aspirations', show that leaders at their personal best were able to challenge the process, inspire a shared vision, enable others to act, model the way, and encourage the heart. Ulrich, *et al.*[14] classify their leadership competences under the following sub-headings: set direction, mobilise individual commitment, engender organisational capability and demonstrate personal character. The lists are numerous, and they lay out the key leadership characteristics. Although there is little benefit to be gained in producing all of them, or even any more of them, in this chapter there are two key messages that emerge in most lists. The messages are well worth considering. First, most of the lists will contain common key elements such as vision, values, integrity, communication, determination or energy, and as such are readily transferable for the leader who operates in any healthcare organisation. The second key message is that many of the leadership capabilities are employer specific, and the lists show how essential it is to know what list is valued by one's employer or prospective employer. Experience will also have taught the experienced leader that a published list of leadership capabilities will often differ from the qualities actually revered in a specific healthcare setting. In my work with leaders, from various sectors, I find it helpful to summarise this by saying to them that leadership has to be contextualised – that is, it has to be sensitive to the needs of the moment and the culture of the organisation; and it has to be personalised – it has to be suitable to the individual's personality. I had been using those two terms for some time before I came across the excellent website of the MIT Leadership Center (http://mitleadership.mit.edu). After describing the nature of leadership they make the point that leaders also need, what they call, a change signature:

> Each person's change signature, like a fingerprint, is unique. Each person brings his/her unique values, skills, experience, tactics, and personality to the role of leader. Each person has his/her personal way of making change happen, although there certainly are patterns across individuals.

2 Leadership is not the same as management

Many writers highlight the difference between management and leadership, and for me the best writer on the subject is John Kotter.[15] Drawing on a classical understanding of management he shows that management concerns itself with planning and budgeting, organising and staffing, and controlling and problem solving, whereas leadership concerns itself with establishing direction, aligning people (communicating the direction), and motivating and inspiring.

Although I agree with Kotter's differentiation, and see it as an important part of understanding leadership, I must also issue a word of caution. I have seen more senior healthcare people sacked for their lack of management of an organisation, usually manifested by an absence of control or corporate governance, than I have seen sacked for a lack of leadership. Cautious managers are at a premium, and visionary leaders are sometimes seen as a dangerous commodity. Different times and different places call for different types of people to head a department or hospital and there seems to be much merit in a healthcare organisation having leaders who can manage and managers who can lead.

On the question of the need for a balance between the need to be a leader and the need to be a manager, I am rather taken with Mintzberg's observation that: 'Management without leadership is sterile; leadership without management is disconnected and encourages hubris'.[16]

3 Leadership is only practised when you have followers

This principle, based on the work of the legendary Peter Drucker,[17] is an important point. Drucker shows that some of the leaders whom he encountered were excruciatingly vain and others were self-effacing to a fault, some were austere and others were ostentatious and pleasure-loving, but all of the effective leaders he knew or observed knew four simple things – they had followers, they achieved results, they set examples and they took responsibility.

Drucker is a managerial and organisation seer of our time, and anyone who questions his view really runs the risk of being a 'fool rushing in where angels fear to tread', but this extract from his writing on leadership does give some cause for concern. A view that leadership is somehow just associated with having followers causes a difficulty for managers and other professionals, who will immediately exclaim 'But Hitler had followers'. They want the definition to contain a moral dimension, otherwise they will believe that the definition is concerned with securing followers at any cost. Who said that healthcare leaders do not have a finely tuned moral perspective! The second concern raised by Drucker's view is that it can be interpreted as seeing leadership as being concerned solely with results. Most people have worked with these so-called leaders. They have achieved *great things*, when measured against the bottom line, but they may also have been nigh on impossible to work for and most people could not wait to leave their organisation. A view of leadership that concentrates on results without looking at the other attributes that bring loyalty and respect seems to run the risk of being considered lopsided and an unhealthy view of leadership. The disciples of Drucker would, with justification, point to the rest of his leadership definition and his library of writings to defend the great man, and any sustained criticism of him would evaporate.

The principle of 'followership' is an important dimension of leadership. The winners of the McKinsey Prize for the best *Harvard Business Review* article in 2000 were the British academics Robert Goffee and Gareth Jones.[18] They asked the fundamental question of executives 'Why would anyone want to be led by you?' over 10 years in dozens of organisations in the USA and Europe. The question would often frighten the leaders as they realised '. . . you can't do anything in organisations without followers, and followers in these "empowered" times are hard to find . . .'. The focus of their research was on leaders 'who excel at inspiring people' and they discovered that these individuals had four qualities.

➤ They selectively showed their weaknesses to emphasise their approachability.

➤ They used intuition to judge their actions.
➤ They employed 'tough empathy' to manage employees.
➤ They capitalised on unique aspects of themselves . . .

Goffee and Jones claim that an individual might find him- or herself in the top position in an organisation, but that without these four essential qualities few people would want to be led by that person. It is important to note that their theory deals with qualities of leadership and the attraction of followers, and not with the achievement of results *per se*. The article and book are well worth reading and studying, and are extremely relevant to the world of health-care. The impact that followers can have on leaders, and the way in which a person's leadership style can be affected by the type of follower, is developed further in Barbara Kellerman's book *Followership*.[19] In my work with leaders they have found it helpful to consider the leadership needed to respond to the five categories of followers identified in Kellerman's typology: Isolate, Bystander, Participant, Activist, Diehard.

4 Leadership is to be found at all levels of the organisation

A serious examination of any organisation will detect leadership taking place in many forms – at the top, in individual departments or wards, and from those who as a part of their role act across the organisation, uniting otherwise potentially disparate parts. Peter Senge[20] classifies what he calls the interplay between three types of leader . . .

➤ *Local line leaders* – 'people with accountability for results', such as ward sisters.
➤ *Internal networkers or community builders* – 'nurturing broad networks of alliances with other like-minded individuals and to help local leaders. They are "seed carriers" of new ideas and practices . . .'
➤ *Executive leaders* – those with 'overall accountability for organisational performance', such as medical and nursing directors and chief executives.

This recognition that leadership exists at all levels of the organisation, and not just in the corridors near the hospital headquarters or wherever, is of paramount importance as it dictates the very approach that is taken to the development of leadership, the style of management practice in the organisation and the recognition that is given to people for their contribution. Yet far too many senior managers and policy makers still refer to an organisation's leaders as if they are to be found only at the top of the pyramidal organisational structure.

5 Leadership is concerned with delivering results

One of my favourite methods of explaining leadership is based on the work of Dave Ulrich, Jack Zenger and Norm Smallwood.[21] In their book *Results-Based Leadership*, they set out a formula for understanding leadership and the balance between the attributes that a leader needs to possess and the results that he or she needs to deliver:

> Being capable and possessing the attributes of leadership is terrific, but capability

must be put to appropriate, purposeful use. Our message to leaders may be put into the simple formula *Effective leadership = attributes × results*. This equation suggests that leaders must strive for excellence in both terms; that is, they must both demonstrate attributes and achieve results.

They then go on to show how this formula can be given scores and how the scores can ascertain leadership effectiveness. This seems eminently sensible and resonates with the experience of most healthcare leaders and managers. Most of them can tell stories about leaders who had it all in terms of attributes, but who could not deliver results and, similarly, leaders who delivered results but who were hated (not too strong a word when one hears the stories of intimidation experienced by them) by their so-called followers.

CASE STUDY 1.1

An article[22] on Steve Ballmer, the Microsoft president and chief executive officer, provides a fascinating insight into the role of a leader. In response to journalist Kim Fletcher's question 'But what does a businessman with his power actually do?', this is what Ballmer said:

> Number one is strategy. Where shall we go? What are the big trends? How do we allocate our research and development resources? I'm not saying you just sit there in your office – oh, lah di dah, what's our strategy? But that's where your energy is consumed.
>
> Number two is being the best possible evangelist for our company, whether it is talking to customers or stockbrokers. I'm not really the number one sales person. I never thought I was very good at that. It's also not my job. My job is to evangelise what we are doing.
>
> Number three is evangelism internally. You've got to do that same job of telling the story, the vision, getting people organised. The last is a responsibility to keep an eye on the controls. Are your revenues and expenses in balance? And then set a culture: what kind of people do we want to have?

One does not have to subscribe to the Microsoft view of the world to recognise the value of pondering on Ballmer's words. What does leadership mean to you? Where do you spend the greatest part of your time? What are your priorities? Can you improve your performance?

CASE STUDY 1.2[23]

In September 2000, 12 identical yachts commenced 'the world's toughest yacht race' – the BT global challenge. Each team set out to race around the globe, one of the toughest feats of teamwork, leadership and human endurance in the modern world.

Academics Cranwell-Ward, Bacon and Mackie decided to track the leadership and performance of the skippers and teams, and this provided them with powerful and pragmatic lessons for leaders working in today's business environment. In their excellent book, they take current leadership theory and issues facing leaders today and synthesise them into a work of benefit to leaders in all walks of life.

Among other things, their work identified a list of personal attributes, management skills and leadership characteristics that the skippers needed in order to be effective. The leadership list is highly informative, and includes purpose, vision, values, recognition, a performance focus, distributed leadership, humour and fun.

FOUR COMPLEMENTARY FACTORS CONCERNING LEADERSHIP

As if my five *negative* and five *positive* principles of leadership were not enough, there are also four other complementary factors to be taken into account to determine how leadership should be exercised within healthcare. They are based on my extensive work with senior managers and clinicians, and these points actually helped my former colleagues to make sense of leadership and the development they needed for themselves.

Emotional intelligence

The *first* factor is the idea of emotional intelligence popularised by the work of Daniel Goleman.[24] Goleman, in his seminal *Harvard Business Review* article, recounts:

> Every businessperson knows a story about a highly intelligent, highly skilled executive who was promoted into a leadership position only to fail at the job. And they also know a story about someone with solid – but not extraordinary – intellectual abilities and technical skills who was promoted into a similar position and then soared.

He goes on to explain that his research found that 'the most effective leaders are alike in one crucial way: they all have a high degree of . . . emotional intelligence,' and he shows that emotional intelligence is the 'sine qua non of leadership'.

As Goleman develops his persuasive argument, he discusses the analysis of his findings and the dramatic result that:

> when I calculated the ratio of technical skills, IQ and emotional intelligence as ingredients of excellent performance, emotional intelligence proved to be twice as important as the others for jobs at all levels.

This is a profoundly important point, and Goleman's claim that emotional intelligence is twice as important as the other factors has a major bearing on anyone's understanding of leadership characteristics.

Goleman shows the five components of emotional intelligence under the headings of self-awareness, self-regulation, motivation, empathy and social skill.

He also shows that it is possible to learn to be more emotionally intelligent. In his later work, *Primal Leadership*, written with Boyatzis and McKee,[25] in a chapter entitled 'The Neuroanatomy of Leadership', he shows how the emotional intelligence domains can be linked to associate leadership competencies.

The importance of this work cannot be over-emphasised, and was even attested by a group of psychiatrists and psychologists whom I once coached on leadership development. To gain such attestation is a rare feat indeed. These clinical directors fully supported the notion. Despite Goleman's work, some healthcare organisations continue to appoint senior leaders on the basis of intelligence or technical ability alone, although it is encouraging to note that selection processes are changing, with many assessment centres paying far more attention to Goleman's work. However, the level of ignorance surrounding his work – or perhaps it is avoidance or apathy rather than ignorance – is still a cause for some concern.

Transformational and transactional leadership

The *second* complementary factor is the significance of transformational and transactional leadership. Much has been written on this subject, and the word 'transformational' in particular has unfortunately entered the management lexicon of clichés. This really is unfortunate, as Bass's[26] work on transformational leadership has a critically important message. He argues that 'transformational leaders . . . behave in ways to achieve superior results by employing one or more of the four components of transformational leadership'. His four components are charismatic leadership (or idealised influence), inspirational motivation, intellectual stimulation and individualised consideration. Bass compares the transformational leadership style with what he calls transactional leadership, and he introduces the concept of positive and negative contingent reinforcement, through the seductive headings of Contingent Reward and Management-by-Exception, and then a third category of Laissez-Faire Leadership.

Bass demonstrates the benefits of transformational leadership, but he also makes the point that there are circumstances in which transactional leadership may be needed. His work is worth studying and has formed an important basis for some of Kouzes and Posner's work, as well as that of other eminent leadership writers. However, Bass's words have also been misused to describe a dynamic style of leadership within an organisation when in reality it may be the very last thing that is actually needed or wanted. It sounds impressive for a healthcare organisation to declare that they require transformational leaders – men and women with vision who will transform the way in which healthcare is delivered, who will bring excellence to every initiative undertaken and so on. The reality is that many healthcare organisations may actually see these transformational leaders – the very people they claim they need – as a 'dangerous breed', and what they actually want are transactional leaders (also known as managers in their minds) who will not take risks, who will be a safe pair of hands, and who will not cause alarm in an ultra-conservative and cautious boardroom.

I once attended an annual conference where Sir Alan Langlands, the Department of Health-based NHS chief executive, in his annual address, raised the issue of the importance of transformational leadership. This is what the NHS needed, he argued, and for 20 minutes or so he gave a magnificent, informative and eloquent speech on the theme of transformational leadership. In the last two or three minutes of his speech Sir Alan turned to three key objectives that the NHS was facing. To say that these were highly operational issues, such as Accident and Emergency waiting times and winter emergency admissions, is not to exaggerate. I noticed the number of NHS chief executives who, at this point in his speech, pulled out of their jacket pockets a piece of paper to note down his three operational points. When I asked them later why this had happened, I was told in no uncertain terms that the chief executives believed that those three points, and not the 20 or so minutes on transformational leadership, would be the issues on which their annual performance and therefore their future careers would be judged. Whether they were right I do not know, but I suspect that they were.

'Situational leadership'

The *third* complementary factor concerns the use of different leadership styles with different people, during different challenges and for different circumstances. The application of a single leadership approach in each and every setting is likely to cause problems of inflexibility, so there is a need to acquire the skill of adapting one's leadership style to meet the different requirements as they present themselves.

Most people will have heard of the term *situational leadership*, which describes the need to adapt one's style of leadership. Blanchard, *et al.*[27] describe four basic styles of leadership as directing (providing specific instructions), coaching (mainly encouraging progress), supporting (facilitating and sharing responsibility with subordinates) and delegating (turning over responsibility). Sometimes this is summarised as: telling, selling, participating, and delegating. Blanchard's work has often been criticised by academics for its populist and parabolic style, but his writings always ring true with the experiences of clinicians and managers who are engaged in the work of leadership.

Bloch and Whiteley[28] appear to go two better than Blanchard as they believe that they have identified six leadership styles, namely authoritative leadership, coaching, democratic leadership, affiliative leadership, pace-setting and a coercive style.

Both of these taxonomies are useful for leaders, as they are illustrative of the issues surrounding leadership style and thus encourage leaders to consider the merits and demerits of different styles for the challenges and people that they encounter in their daily task of leading a healthcare organisation. They are also the perfect way in which to answer the soldier, the surgeon and the barrister who will always ask the disingenuous question, 'Do you really expect me to be participative in my leadership style when I am trying to kill the enemy (soldier) / save a life (surgeon) / keep someone out of jail (barrister)?' The question, disingenuous or not, is the perfect invitation to discuss leadership style in a highly practical way.

Twenty-first-century challenges

The fourth and final complementary factor concerns leading amidst the challenges of the twenty-first century. The world of the twenty-first century will be different. We know this with certainty because the changes associated with the twenty-first century started happening in the 1980s and 1990s – they did not suddenly spring into existence at midnight on 31 December 1999. As a result, wise healthcare managers have been adapting their leadership styles gradually to meet the new challenges. The new world of organisations will require, according to Bennis and Nanus's classic work:[29]

> leaders at every level and fewer managers; leading by vision where new directions are created for long-term business growth; more collegial organisations; empowering and inspiring individuals, and also facilitating teamwork; the leader as coach, who creates learning organisations; the leader as change agent, who evolves the culture; and the leader who is also responsible for developing future leaders, and serving as a leader of leaders.

This fourth complementary factor will also encompass three quite specific leadership challenges among those who are the followers, namely the ever-increasing challenge with regard to the leadership of professionals, the leadership of what has been termed 'generations X and Y', and the rise of the typically unassuming and authentic leader.

The first issue will be familiar to those who lead teams of doctors, nurses or other professionals. You will know that conventional leadership principles sometimes do not work, and the problem does not lie with the leader but with the fact that professionals, of whatever discipline, usually do not want to be managed. They are professionals, proud of their education and professionalism, independent in their thinking, and wanting as much freedom as possible to practise their noble art. In *First Among Equals*[30] the challenge of leading professionals is highlighted and will surely cause any experienced leader to nod in agreement:

> Certain characteristics of professionals that allow them to do their jobs effectively create barriers to them being successful in the group setting. Most professionals are trained to be sceptical and will almost always critically challenge any new idea, bringing to bear their analytical gifts. Getting agreement on even the smallest issues can be tough.

The second challenge concerns the leadership of the so-called generation X and generation Y. These are those people who do not share the view of the world that sits comfortably with the baby-boomers born in the decade after World War Two. This challenge has to do with the tricky issue of age. Any leader will know that the beliefs and attitudes of those born after around 1970 and those born in the 1950s are very different, and most people occupying senior positions of leadership are closer (in attitude if not in age) to the baby-boomers. This is why there is often a problem in basic communication – values and aspirations are significantly different. How often have you heard a senior nurse or doctor declare 'It wasn't like that in my day!'? Bennis and Thomas, in their entertaining book *Geeks and Geezers*[31] (two American slang words for the under-30s and the over-50s), help leaders to think deeply about people who see the world quite differently, and this type of thinking has already become an imperative for most leaders.

The factors that influence the development of generation X, according to a working paper for the think-tank Demos by David Cannon,[32] include the following:

➤ invasive media – where information is required at a fast rate
➤ the 'global' generation – they wear global products, have travelled extensively, and think of global issues
➤ accessible communications and computer tools – they communicate differently
➤ new attitudes – demonstrated by a decline in trust, and a belief in self-reliance, independence and choice.

The attitudes of generation Y, according to Cannon, are significantly different from those of generation X and so place quite different challenges before leaders. Generation Y qualities and values are likely to include the following:

➤ they are motivated and goal orientated
➤ they need regular reinforcement
➤ they are technologically wise
➤ they like to work in teams
➤ they are good at multi-tasking.

The third challenge sounds as if it borders on the contradictory, and it probably does. There is evidence that many organisations are appointing chief executives who, to use Maccoby's[33] phrase, are narcissistic leaders. According to Maccoby:

> this love of the limelight often stems from their personalities . . . that is both good and bad news: narcissists are good for organisations that need people with vision and the courage to take them in new directions. But narcissists can also lead organisations into trouble by refusing to listen to the advice and warnings of their managers.

Those words seem particularly prescient as we reflect on the financial sector and the calamitous performance of certain banks in 2009.

Standing in contradistinction to the narcissistic tendencies of some leaders is the evidence in Collins' best-selling work, *Good to Great*[34] that the building of a great organisation can be done best by what he calls *level 5 leaders*. These are leaders who have a *professional will* and a *personal humility* that is typically modest, quiet and calm, who are organisationally not self-focused, and who praise other people. One of the unexpected findings of his work was that:

> larger-than-life, celebrity leaders who ride in from the outside are negatively correlated with (organisations) going from good to great. Ten of eleven good-to-great

CEOs came from inside the organisation, whereas the comparison organisations tried outside CEOs six times more often.

In similar vein, Bill George, the former chairman and CEO of Medtronic, makes the case for leaders who are authentic. His first best-selling book *Authentic Leadership – Rediscovering the Secrets to Creating Lasting Value*[35] 'persuasively demonstrates that authentic leaders of mission-driven companies will create far greater shareholder value than financially oriented companies'. And George knows what he is talking about: under his leadership, Medtronic's market capitalisation soared from $1.1 billion to $60 billion in a 12-year period. The great message of the book is captured in the title of the first chapter – leadership is authenticity, not style – where he contends that authentic leaders demonstrate five qualities: understanding their purpose; practising solid values; leading with heart; establishing connected relationships; and demonstrating self-discipline. In George's subsequent book, *True North*,[36] he sets out to help leaders to discover their authentic leadership. His premise is that

> [j]ust as a compass points toward a magnetic field, your True North pulls you toward the purpose of your leadership. When you follow your internal compass, your leadership will be authentic, and people will naturally want to associate with you.

He goes on to explain five key areas under the headings of: knowing your authentic self; defining your values and leadership principles; understanding your motivations; building your support team; and, staying grounded by integrating all aspects of your life.

Collins's and George's work have many implications for recruitment and selection, succession planning and, within the scope of this chapter, the leadership style that one should adopt.

Anyone placing the work of Maccoby, Collins and George side by side may be faced with something of a dilemma. However, the search for an appropriate leadership style to develop in a healthcare organisation, through the efforts of the chief executive and the entire leadership team at all levels in the organisation, needs to be informed by a wide range of considerations. Only then can the right approach(es) be developed and the hospital and its people led to the proper ends.

As the next-but-one section will show, I am convinced that the principles of servant-leadership should be one of the major leadership philosophies to be examined carefully by all healthcare organisations.

LEADERSHIP AND THE PATIENT EXPERIENCE

So far in this chapter, I have defined leadership by saying what it is and what it isn't; emphasised its significance and stressed that it has to be viewed within certain contexts and must be personalised; I have also linked it to one's values through the notion of being authentic; and, expressly and implicitly, shown that leadership has to be connected to the 'bottom line' of the organisation.

Logically that raises a crucial question that anyone in healthcare will wish to ask and which I ask firmly wearing my patient's hat: what evidence exists to support the notion that leadership and the development of leadership practice actually improves the lot of the patient? A health-service client commissioned me to explore that very question and my findings were turned into a 15 000-word monograph, which the *British Journal of Healthcare Management* published in 2009.[37]

The first thing to say is that the evidence is not plentiful (and I suggest this should be a beneficial area for future researchers to explore), but evidence does exist in quantitative and qualitative form. I subdivided my findings into what I called: peer reviewed journal articles; professional journals; the work of healthcare regulators and clinical professional bodies; the publications of the Institute of Healthcare Improvement; publications from other public and private sectors; and what I called axiomatic evidence, based on the experience of individuals I interviewed, university faculties and reputable healthcare agencies engaged in leadership development over many decades.

The monograph's seven conclusions should act as an encouragement to further leadership development and also temper those who engage in leadership and its development without sufficient thought. My conclusions, in the briefest form, were the following.

1 The evidence, whilst not voluminous, is sufficient to assert that effective leadership does have a positive impact on the patient experience.

2 Further research into the sometimes indecipherable links between leadership development and the patient experience is welcome.

3 Central to the use of the term *effective leadership development* is a commitment to on-going evaluation and validation of initiatives.

4 It is essential to establish robust return on investment (ROI) criteria and report them to the satisfaction of all parties.

5 It is important to use the experience of credible leadership development practitioners, who can demonstrate a link between the development intervention and significant improvements for patient care.

6 There is a need to keep under review the nature and practice of leadership within an evolving healthcare world and to encourage a greater role for clinicians.

7 The central message for policy makers is that, wherever possible, effective leadership development should be given higher priority.

SERVANT-LEADERSHIP

The notion of the leader as servant was originally given prominence in the twentieth century through the writings of Robert Greenleaf.[38] His central thesis was that 'caring for persons, the more able and the less able serving each other, is the rock upon which a good society is built . . . [and] one way that some people serve is to lead'. This became his inspiration and the driving force behind his belief that leadership should be based on the concept of the leader being *primus inter pares* – the first among equals. This belief resulted in a series of challenging essays, speeches and articles that have stood the test of time. His essays are not the easiest of reads – he was in many ways a philosopher and polemicist – but the following examples of quotes from his work help to illustrate his ideas:

> The great leader is seen as servant first.
> The only authority deserving one's allegiance is that which is freely and knowingly granted by the led.
> Do those served grow as persons? Do they become healthier, wiser, freer, more autonomous, more likely themselves to become servants?
> Better performance for the public good.
> Leaders do not elicit trust unless one has confidence in their values and competence and unless they have a sustaining spirit that will support the tenacious pursuit of a goal.
> I am in the business of growing people.

Even with quotes such as these one is grateful to Larry Spears, the former Chief Executive of the Greenleaf Center for Servant-Leadership in Indianapolis and now CEO of the eponymous centre, for presenting the key principles of servant-leadership as a set of 10 characteristics.

The 10 characteristics of the servant-leader[39] (substantially abbreviated)

1 *Listening*: '. . . a deep commitment to listening intently to others . . . They seek to listen receptively to what is being said (and not being said!). Listening also involves getting in touch with one's own inner voice . . . listening, coupled with regular periods of reflection, is essential to the growth of the servant-leader.'

2 *Empathy*: '. . . striving to understand and empathise with others. People need to be accepted and recognised for their special and unique spirits. One must assume the good intentions of co-workers and not reject them as people, even when forced to reject their behaviour or performance.'

3 *Healing*: 'Learning to heal is a powerful force for transformation and integration. One of the great strengths of servant-leadership is the potential for healing one's self and others . . . servant-leaders recognise that they have an opportunity to help make whole those with whom they come in contact.'

4 *Awareness*: 'General awareness, and especially self-awareness, strengthens the servant-leader . . . Awareness . . . aids in understanding issues involving ethics and values. It enables one to view most situations from a more integrated position.'

5 *Persuasion*: '. . . a reliance upon persuasion, rather than positional authority, in making decisions within an organisation . . . the servant-leader is effective at building consensus within groups.'

6 *Conceptualisation*: 'Servant-leaders seek to nurture their abilities to "dream great dreams" . . . The ability to look at a problem . . . from a conceptualising perspective means that one must think beyond day-to-day realities . . . a manager who wishes to be a servant-leader must stretch his or her thinking to encompass broader-based conceptual thinking.'

7 *Foresight*: 'The ability to foresee the likely outcome of a situation is hard

to define, but easy to identify . . . Foresight is a characteristic that enables servant-leaders to understand the lessons from the past, the realities of the present, and the likely consequence of a decision for the future. It is deeply rooted within the intuitive mind.'

8 *Stewardship:*[40] '. . . [means] "holding something in trust for another". Robert Greenleaf's view of all institutions was one in which CEOs, staff, directors and trustees all played significant roles in holding their institutions in trust for the greater good of society.'

9 *Commitment to the growth of people:* '. . . people have an intrinsic value beyond their tangible contributions as workers. As such, servant-leaders are deeply committed to the personal, professional and spiritual growth of each and every individual within the institution.'

10 *Building community:* '. . . servant-leaders seek to identify a means for building community among those who work within a given institution.'

Although the language can sound sentimental at times, and certainly appears to be out of kilter with the tough-sounding world of performance management, there is a hard edge to the concept. Robert Greenleaf wrote: 'The servant as leader always empathises, always accepts the person, but sometimes refuses to accept some of the person's effort or performance as good enough . . .' Adopting the characteristics of a servant-leader and then applying them in our healthcare organisations is difficult, and I would not claim to have mastered all of these characteristics sufficiently well to offer authoritative advice on how to implement them in every part of the healthcare network. However, I am more than prepared to express my belief in servant-leadership and to explain how I came to be committed to its principles. The following passages are based on a speech I delivered at the Greenleaf Servant-Leadership Conference in London in November 2002.

BOX 1.1 A personal journey: 'I remain, sir, your obedient servant'

Most of the great religions of the world reserve a special place in their heart for the convert, especially those converts who have come to faith somewhat late in life. The convert's stumbling discovery of the truth is celebrated and encouraged. Obvious gaps in knowledge, and sometimes these gaps amount to alarming chasms, are glossed over with benign and understanding smiles, and their very words, their testimony, are an encouragement to those who have practised and studied the faith for decades, if not generations.

I do not want to suggest that servant-leadership is a religion, to be compared with Christianity, Judaism, Islam or some other faith, but I will suggest later that there is an inspirational, even spiritual dimension to the writings and work on servant-leadership. Neither will I claim that you come to a belief in servant-leadership through faith, but I do believe that the metaphor of a convert is an apt description of the journey I have been on for the best part of 30 years. By using the metaphor I also wish to invoke a certain sympathy in my audience: I am a relatively new convert and the gaps in my knowledge will soon be clear for all to see. So I look to you, those experienced 'in the faith', to celebrate even my stumbling discoveries, to gloss over my serious omissions with benign smiles, and to be encouraged that someone such as I has discovered the truth of servant-leadership, at last.

It is important for me to say something about my career to date. Since October 2001 I have been a professor of leadership and organisation development. Prior to that I worked as a chief executive within the National Health Service, and I have worked in the manufacturing sector, where I specialised in industrial relations. The job titles I held at various times are of little importance as they are mere labels that organisations, mainly for their benefit, hang on a person. What is far more important is that in each and every job I was passionately committed (one boss even called me a zealot) to the people of the organisation and to the way in which they were developed. In some jobs it was easier to demonstrate that fact and in others, especially those concerned with the hurly-burly of industrial relations, it was much harder, if not impossible.

Throughout my working life I have made sure that my reading and academic studies have supported this commitment to people and their development. So you can imagine the joy I felt when I came across the writings of Robert Greenleaf, Larry Spears and many others on servant-leadership, and the complementary work of people like Max DePree. What surprised me most of all is that their books had not landed on my desk much earlier. After reading them, I felt very much like M Jourdain, one of Molière's characters, who in a discussion with a professor of philosophy made a great discovery and exclaimed 'Good heavens! For more than forty years I have been speaking prose without knowing it'. My experience was similar.

As I read the books and reflected on them, four main arguments emerged that convinced me of the merits of servant-leadership. I wish to look at each of these four arguments and encourage you to continue your reflection on this most important of areas.

Inspirational evidence

The first argument I shall call the *inspirational evidence*. If you are a bibliophile, like me, then you can't go for many weeks without buying a book. My study shelves are straining under the weight of the leadership, learning and development books I have bought (and read!) in the past few years. Some of the books are acknowledged classics in the field, others are little gems which one day will achieve classic status and some, I have to confess, are unlikely to be opened ever again. On my bookshelves are authors whose writings I almost revere – people like Peter Senge, Warren Bennis, Arie De Geus, Rosabeth Moss Kanter and many, many others. As I read the books I noticed that time and again I would come across phrases such as these:

> For many years I have told people that although there are a lot of books on leadership, there is only one that serious students have to read – *Servant-Leadership* by Robert K Greenleaf . . . few [other books] penetrate to deeper insights into the nature of real leadership . . . [Greenleaf] says that the first and most important choice a leader makes is the choice to serve, without which one's capacity to lead is profoundly limited. That choice is not an action in the normal sense – it's not something you do, but an expression of your being.[41]

. . . I am a fan of Robert Greenleaf and think that servant-leadership is the foundation for effective leadership . . .[42]

. . . servant-leadership is the enabling art to accomplishing any worthy objective.[43]

This is a wonderful book [referring to *Leadership is an Art* by Max DePree] . . . it says more about leadership . . . than many of the much longer books that have been published on the subject.[44]

I could quote many other examples, but I hope these few quotations will illustrate my first argument. The writings of Robert Greenleaf, and the concept of servant-leadership, have impressed and had a profound effect on many of those people who are, in this generation, seen as leading authorities in their field.

On a personal level, I found the writings to be inspirational. I had to find out more.

Business case

My second argument is the *business case*. There is always a danger in illustrating a glowing example of a certain principle. Peters and Waterman found that out after they launched their seminal work *In Search of Excellence!*[45] No sooner had they extolled the excellence virtues of particular companies than some of those very organisations went into decline – terminal decline in certain instances (not that this had anything to do with Peters and Waterman, of course). However, the principles that they discovered stood the test of time and have become an accepted part of management theory.

The same, I believe, is true of servant-leadership. I know little about TD Industries, Southwest Airlines, Synovus Financial Corporation, Herman Miller Inc., The Container Store, and the other oft-quoted examples of servant-leadership in action, but you would have to possess the head-in-the-sand qualities of an ostrich to ignore the evidence from these organisations. It is surely no coincidence that these organisations often score well in the list of best organisations to work for, so in a sense their employees provide proof of the business case, alongside the financial evidence. To pay no attention to the various pieces of evidence seems to me to commit the folly of our forefathers who ignored the total quality revolution occurring in the Far East until it was almost too late.

Although I confess to being intrigued by new '-isms' in the world of organisations and their development, it has to be recognised that the concept of servant-leadership is not some new idea or passing fad, but something that has stood the test of time.

Moral case

The *moral case* is my third argument. Throughout my working life I have been appalled by the manner in which some managers have treated their employees. It seems that Henry Ford's alleged comment, 'Why is it that whenever I ask for a pair of hands, a brain comes attached?', is alive and well in far too many companies. I clearly remember my first experience of this. When I started work in the manufacturing sector I met a man whom I shall call David Jackson. He worked, I learned to my dismay, as a sweeper. He spent all day brushing up the mess left by other workers. Yet this man was a respected pillar of his community, someone whom people looked up to, someone who could be relied upon for his wisdom and judgement, and someone who exercised valuable leadership within his church.

Max DePree memorably addresses this very principle in *Leadership is an Art*[46] by quoting the poet Thomas Gray to lament the fact that 'talent may go unnoticed and unused':

> Full many a gem of purest ray serene
> The dark unfathomed caves of ocean bear:
> Full many a flower is born to blush unseen
> And waste its sweetness on the desert air.

I know that servant-leadership is not a philanthropic movement established to liberate all and sundry from every menial task, but the reason David Jackson's qualities were not used by that company was due to a senior management belief that 'manual grades' had little if anything to offer the organisation. I believe that we have a moral duty to treat people with respect – to make use of the potential within them, to develop their contribution, to see them as 'partners' within the organisation (the word 'partners' is used in the stakeholder sense of the word), and to realise that serving their interests is consistent with serving the needs of the organisation.

I cannot emphasise this moral point too much. Recently, I read the autobiography of Jack Welch,[47] the former CEO of General Electric, whom *Fortune* called the greatest manager of the twentieth century. The book is an exciting tale of how he transformed the performance of the company, a highly commendable act, and it stands as a textbook to be read by anyone interested in the role of management. However, it is also clear why he inherited the sobriquet 'Neutron Jack' as he purged the organisation of layer after layer of management. He would seize any concept to improve the bottom-line performance of the company (many commendable actions in my view), and no doubt he would have taken hold of the concept of servant-leadership also if someone had shown him that it would improve profitability. But that misses the point as far as I am concerned. Whilst there is a business case argument for servant-leadership, to apply the concept without any recognition of the moral imperative shows little understanding of its key principles.

Evidence from human nature

My fourth and final argument is the *evidence from human nature*. I can sum up this point in three words by saying, 'Because people respond!' People are amazing, and they constantly surprise others, and themselves, by what they are able to achieve if allowed to operate under appropriate conditions. I could tell story after story of people who appear to 'grow' before your very eyes when placed in the right environment. What is true for individuals is also true for groups of people, and is also true for organisations as a whole. But with organisations it is much harder. It seems that senior people find it hard to believe that what they know to be true for individuals, and have seen happening for groups, can also be used to transform their organisation.

From principle to practice

So there you have it, the four main reasons why I am pleased to associate myself with servant-leadership – the inspirational evidence, the business case, the moral case and the evidence from human nature.

However, coming to terms with the principles of servant-leadership has not been plain sailing. Along the way I have encountered and have had to tackle a number of misunderstandings.

The first misunderstanding was all my own work! I have to confess that the first time I read Robert Greenleaf's book I thought it to be a rather sentimental work. Whilst I warmed to his affirmation that 'I am in the business of growing people – people who are stronger, healthier, more autonomous, more self-reliant, more competent . . .', I was puzzled by the almost off-hand way in which he added, 'Incidentally, we also make and sell at a profit things that people want to buy so we can pay for all of this'. It appealed to the cavalier spirit within me, but I found little in it to fit in with the 'real world', and it would have been impossible to convince my hard-nosed health colleagues to try to apply such principles. However, the notions contained in his words 'one way that some people serve is to lead' and his view of society where 'the more able serve the less able' were tantalisingly attractive propositions.

The reason for my misunderstanding is that I failed to understand that servant-leadership is not an alternative, quasi-New Age system where the needs of people are paramount and 'bottom-line' performance is of little relevance, or a coincidental outcome of treating staff decently and with dignity. As I read other writers it dawned on me that servant-leadership and organisational efficiency and sound management practice were not mutually exclusive concepts. For this insight I am grateful to people such as:

- Max DePree,[48] who wrote '. . . liberating people to do what is required of them in the most effective and humane way possible . . .'
- Ken Blanchard[49] who, in correcting someone's misunderstanding of servant-leadership, wrote '. . . their assumption when they heard the term was that managers should be working for their people, who would be deciding what to do, when to do it, and how to do it. If that was what servant-leadership was all about, it didn't sound to them like leadership at all. It sounded more like the inmates were running the prison. I think it's important for us to correct this misconception. Leadership has two aspects – a visionary part and an implementation part . . .'
- Larry Spears,[50] who showed that '. . . servant-leadership emphasises increased service to others, a holistic approach to work, building a sense of community, and the sharing of power in decision making'.

These writers recognised that there are times in all organisations when hard decisions have to be taken and when employees are shown clearly what they are expected to deliver. Servant-leadership did not contradict the basic rigours of management, but influenced the way in which management activities were conducted.

(Before I leave this point, let me say something in parentheses. It strikes me that the more one delves into this area, the more one finds other thinkers, on the meaning of work and organisations, expressing similar notions. Some support the principles – without necessarily using the term servant-leadership – because they see them as reflecting how human nature at its best is constructed, a human nature designed to be able to reach beyond itself and to relate to others in communities of service.)

Other misunderstandings were the work of my colleagues. One colleague, a chief executive of an NHS trust, declared that as he was both a public servant and a leader, then obviously he was a servant-leader. Not only did he misunderstand the ethos of servant-leadership, but his leadership practice in that organisation was the very antithesis of the principles espoused by Greenleaf and others. In terms of the traditional boss as opposed to the servant as leader, set out helpfully in McGee-Cooper and Looper's volume,[51] he operated in a highly competitive manner, sometimes used fear and intimidation to get what he wanted, controlled information in order to maintain power, used internal politics for personal gain, and viewed accountability as a means to assign blame. Some servant-leader!

Yet this presents something of a dilemma. On the one hand, you are grateful to anyone who appears to be lending support to your attempts to develop the concept of servant-leadership in your organisation, and especially in the healthcare sector. On the other hand, you are alarmed that his style of management will alienate the people you are trying to influence. What do you do? Tackle the problem head-on and potentially create a hostile environment, or ignore the issue in the hope that the boorish individual will disappear into the undergrowth?

Another manager, who heard me speaking about servant-leadership at a conference, saw it as an opportunity to gain access to what she erroneously believed to be the corridors of power – the NHS trust headquarters. She wanted to develop her career and was continually on the lookout for the latest thinking, any new ideas being discussed by senior management, so that she could use them as a shibboleth to help her career development. With this sort of person any newly heard approach would do as long as it served her short- and medium-term career aspirations. I do not wish to appear harsh in my description of her – in many ways I admire her determination and motivation. But it does raise a further dilemma. There is an understandable temptation to see the concept of servant-leadership as something so important that one has to do all one can to retain the purity of the message (again I am trespassing on the territory of religious belief). At the same time, if one engages in proselytising – spreading the message – then inevitably new adherents may use areas of servant-leadership for their own ends. It's a matter of purity versus popularity.

My final example of misunderstanding is taken from the world of academia. One of my university colleagues appeared to think I had taken leave of my senses and helpfully emailed me a copy of an article written by Russell and Stone, two US academics.[52] In their article they used a forensic approach to question the very foundations of servant-leadership. The article was entertaining, well researched, and an important contribution to the debate showing the importance of stimulating the debate on servant-leadership, of producing further examples of its success, of stimulating research, and of encouraging the emergence of apologists.

The four arguments: in conclusion

For me, all four arguments or reasons for my belief in servant-leadership are fundamentally important and, again for me, I cannot see how the concept can exist and be relevant without all four of them being present.

Firstly, there is a need to appreciate how servant-leadership has inspired other people, especially those people who have had such a profound impact on the development of others. Also, it is essential to allow its inspirational qualities to influence the way in which you practise your own leadership role.

Secondly, there is a need to recognise that successful organisations, whether driven by the concepts of health or social gain, or by profit, are the bedrock upon which much of the remainder of society is founded. Without their contribution, education, health, the arts and much else would be in a parlous state. So servant-leadership is, and should be, inextricably connected to the performance of the organisation.

Thirdly, there is a need to treat people with dignity and respect. Hanging on my office wall is a copy of the International Charter for Human Rights, a powerful reminder of these principles and something that is inherently a part of the servant-leadership message.

Fourthly, there is a need to share experiences of where servant-leadership is working successfully.

Most of you will have recognised that the title I have given this paper, 'I remain, sir, your obedient servant', is taken from the antiquated (and long since departed) style in which various authorities, in many countries, would bring their letters to a close. If any of you received such a letter from the Inland Revenue, the Armed Forces, or some other similar agency, I can understand how you would have pondered the exact meaning of the word 'servant'. But the concept is sound – all of us need to see ourselves as having the privilege of serving others.

My conference speech was delivered in 2002 when, as I admitted at the time, my understanding of servant-leadership was in its infancy. Since then I have developed my understanding and have appreciated becoming involved in the promotion of servant-leadership internationally through board membership of the Greenleaf Centre for Servant-Leadership UK, as a member of the editorial board of the *International Journal for Servant-Leadership*, involvement in the Greenleaf Scholars Program administered through the University of Michigan, and by having the great privilege of writing two books on the subject.[53,54]

CONCLUSION: THE ANATOMY OF A LEADER

To be a leader is a major challenge. It calls for individuals who can paint a picture of a better future and then encourage others to follow them in pursuit of that obtainable dream.

In the past ten years I must have read almost 200 books on the subject of leadership. Some of them have been awe-inspiring and challenging, and others have left me (not to put too fine a point on it) feeling a little disappointed. As I thought about these books, the great ones and the not-so-good ones, I came to the conclusion that the messages in many of them could be recalled through a little human anatomy. What could be more appropriate for a healthcare book? So here, presented somewhat tongue in cheek, is my anatomical and metaphorical guide to leadership.

To be a successful leader there is a need for:

➤ eyes – to see where one is going
➤ mouth – to convince others what needs to be done
➤ ears – to listen to those wiser than oneself
➤ brain – to think and devise appropriate strategies
➤ shoulders – to carry heavy burdens
➤ heart – to possess a passion for the work to be done
➤ nose – to smell out trouble before others spot it
➤ stomach – for an appetite for success, but also the intestinal fortitude ('guts') for the unpleasant jobs
➤ backbone – to make courageous decisions
➤ feet – to lead by walking ahead of the followers and to manage by walking around
➤ knees – to bend in contrition when needing understanding and perhaps forgiveness
➤ hands – to work hard and to punch one's weight
➤ fingers – to point the direction for the business
➤ reproductive organs – to develop successors
➤ soul – to follow one's conscience and values, and use one's will.

Key actions

1 You need to find out the leadership qualities that your healthcare organisation values, and to observe how these qualities are practised by other leaders in different circumstances and with different people.

2 Never fall for the belief that leadership is entirely about being transformational ('the vision thing'), and realise that in healthcare, as in most other organisations, you also need to be a competent manager (transactional).

3 The notion of emotional intelligence is not the latest fad, and understanding the concept and determining your own strengths and weaknesses can substantially help you as a leader.

4 To lead is to serve others. Leadership is a privilege and it should be encouraged wherever it is found, at all levels of the organisation.

REFERENCES

1 Institute of Directors (2002) *Developing Tomorrow's Leaders*. Development Dimensions International, London.

2 Goffee R and Jones G (2009) Proof positive. *People Management*. 18 June: 28–30.

3 Bass BM (1990) *Bass and Stogdill's Handbook of Leadership*. The Free Press, New York.

4 Department of Health website: www.dh.gov.uk/en/News/Recentstories/Dtt_098268 (accessed 22 April 2009).

5 Fuller RM and Goldsmith M (2001) *The Leadership Investment – How The World's Best Organisations Gain Strategic Advantages Through Leadership Development*. American Management Association, New York.

6 Pettigrew A (2001) Does leadership make a difference to organisational performance? *Warwick Business School Nexus Journal*. Autumn issue: 16–18.

7 Grint K (2005) *Leadership: Limits and Possibilities*. Palgrave Macmillan, Hampshire.

8 One of Warren Bennis's many famous quotes – source unknown.

9 Murray Y (2002) Article on Brad Langevad. *The Sunday Times*. 30 June.

10 Maxwell JC (1998) *The 21 Irrefutable Laws of Leadership*. Thomas Nelson, Nashville, TN.

11 Daft RL (2001) *The Leadership Experience*. Harcourt College, Orlando, FL.

12 Goleman D, Boyatzis R and McKee A (2002) *Primal Leadership*. Harvard Business School Press, Boston, MA.

13 Kouzes JM and Posner BZ (1995) *The Leadership Challenge*. Jossey-Bass, San Francisco, CA.

14 Ulrich D, Zenger J and Smallwood N (1999) *Results-Based Leadership*. Harvard Business School Press, Boston, MA.

15 Kotter J (1990) *A Force for Change*. The Free Press, New York.

16 Mintzberg H (2004) *Managers not MBAS*. Pearson Education, Harlow.

17 Drucker P (1996) Foreword. In: *The Leader of the Future*. The Drucker Foundation, Jossey-Bass, San Francisco, CA.

18 Goffee R and Jones G (2000) Why should anyone be led by you? *Harvard Business Review*. September–October: 63–70.

19 Kellerman B (2008) *Followership – How Followers Are Creating Change and Changing Leaders*. Harvard Business, Boston, MA.

20 Senge P (1999) *The Dance of Change*. Currency Doubleday, New York.

21 Ulrich D, Zenger J and Smallwood N (1999) *Results-Based Leadership*. Harvard Business School Press, Boston, MA.

22 Fletcher K (unknown) Interview with Steve Ballmer. *Daily Telegraph Magazine*. 34–6.

23 Cranwell-Ward J, Bacon A and Mackie R (2002) *Inspiring Leadership: staying afloat in turbulent times*. Thomson, London. (The words in the case study are based on the text of their excellent book.)

24 Goleman D (1998) What makes a leader? *Harvard Business Review*. November–December: 93–102.

25 Goleman D, Boyatzis R and McKee A (2002) *Primal Leadership*. Harvard Business School Press, Boston, MA.

26 Bass BM (1998) *Transformational Leadership*. Lawrence Erlbaum Associates, Mahwah, NJ.

27 Blanchard K, Zigarmi P and Zigarmi D (2000) *Leadership and the One-Minute Manager*. HarperCollins Business, London.

28 Bloch S and Whiteley P (2003) *Complete Leadership*. Pearson Education, Harlow.

29 Bennis W and Nanus B (1986) *Leaders: strategies for taking charge*. Harper and Row, New York.

30 McKenna PJ and Maister DH (2002) *First Among Equals*. The Free Press, New York.

31 Bennis WG and Thomas RJ (2002) *Geeks and Geezers*. Harvard Business School Press, Boston, MA.

32 Cannon D (2002) Generation X and the new work ethic. In: J Cranwell-Ward,

A Bacon and R Mackie (eds) *Inspiring Leadership: staying afloat in turbulent times*. Thomson, London.

33 Maccoby M (2002) Narcissistic leaders. In: *Harvard Business Review on What Makes a Leader*. Harvard Business School Press, Boston, MA.

34 Collins J (2001) *Good to Great*. Random House Business Books, London.

35 George B (2003) *Authentic Leadership*. Jossey-Bass, San Francisco, CA.

36 George B (2007) *True North*. Jossey-Bass, San Francisco, CA.

37 Prosser S (2009) Leadership development: does it make a difference? *B J Healthc Manage*. 15(3): 1–29.

38 Greenleaf RK (1977) *Servant-Leadership*. The Paulist Press, New York.

39 Spears LC (1998) Tracing the growing impact of servant-leadership. In: L Spears (ed.) *Insights on Leadership*. John Wiley and Sons, New York.

40 Block P (1996) *Stewardship*. Berrett-Koehler, San Francisco, CA.

41 Senge P (1998) Introduction. In: J Jaworski (ed.) *Synchronicity: the inner path of leadership*. Berrett-Koehler, San Francisco, CA.

42 Blanchard K (2002) Foreword: The heart of servant-leadership. In: LC Spears and M Lawrence (eds) *Focus on Leadership*. John Wiley and Sons, New York.

43 Covey SR (2002) Servant-leadership and community leadership in the twenty-first Century. In: LC Spears and M Lawrence (eds) *Focus on Leadership*. John Wiley and Sons, New York.

44 Drucker PF (1996) Testimonial to M DePree. In: *Leadership is an Art*. Currency Doubleday, New York.

45 Peters T and Waterman R (1982) *In Search of Excellence*. Harper and Row, New York.

46 DePree M (1996) *Leadership is an Art*. Currency Doubleday, New York.

47 Welch J and Byrne JA (2001) *Jack*. Headline, London.

48 DePree M (1996) *Leadership is an Art*. Currency Doubleday, New York.

49 Blanchard K (1998) Servant-leadership revisited. In: LC Spears (ed.) *Insights on Leadership*. John Wiley and Sons, New York.

50 Spears LC (2002) Tracing the past, present and future of servant-leadership. In: LC Spears and M Lawrence (eds) *Focus on Leadership*. John Wiley and Sons, New York.

51 McGee-Cooper A and Looper G (2001) *The Essentials of Servant-Leadership: principles in practice*. Pegasus Communications, Boston, MA.

52 Russell RF and Stone AG (2002) A review of servant-leadership attributes: developing a practical model. *Leadership Organis Dev J*. 23(3): 145–57

53 Prosser S (2007) *To Be A Servant-Leader*. Paulist Press, New Jersey.

54 Prosser S (forthcoming 2010) *You can move Cheese! The Role of an Effective Servant-Leader*. Paulist Press, New Jersey.

CHAPTER 2

Organisation development:
what on earth is it?

'There's glory for you!' 'I don't know what you mean by "glory",' Alice said. 'I meant, "there's a nice knock-down argument for you!"'. 'But "glory" doesn't mean "a nice knock-down argument",' Alice objected. 'When I use a word,' Humpty-Dumpty said in a rather scornful tone, 'it means just what I choose it to mean – neither more nor less.'

Lewis Carroll, *Through the Looking-Glass* (1872)

Organisation development (OD) appears to be one of those concepts that mean different things to different people. Anyone looking through a standard textbook on the subject would see the subtle nuances that differentiate the approach preferred by one practitioner over another, and anyone who has seen OD practitioners in action will know that their interventions are often predicated on their preferences and their understanding of what OD actually means.

The acclaimed writer Warner Burke[1] defines OD as '. . . a process of fundamental change in an organisation's culture,' and French, Bell and Zawacki,[2] authors of a definitive OD textbook, present what appear to be three definitions of OD within the opening paragraph of their book (presumably they would highlight the complementary nature of the definitions):

> OD is the applied behavioural science discipline dedicated to improving organisations and the people in them through the use of the theory and practice of planned change.

Basically, OD is a process for teaching people how to solve problems, take advantage of opportunities, and learn how to do that better and better over time.

> OD is a systematic process for applying behavioural science principles and practices in organisations to increase individual and organisational effectiveness.

Cummings and Worley,[3] authors of another standard OD textbook, see OD as:

a system-wide application of behavioural science knowledge to the planned development, improvement and reinforcement of the strategies, structures and processes that lead to organisation effectiveness.

Helpfully, Cummings and Worley expand their definition to show that:

OD applies to the strategy, structure and processes of an entire system . . . is based on behavioural science knowledge and practice . . . is concerned with managing planned change . . . involves both the creation and the subsequent reinforcement of change . . . [and] is oriented to improving organisational effectiveness . . .

Even Warren Bennis,[4] best known for his writings on leadership, has cast light on the exact meaning of OD by offering the following:

OD is a response to change, a complex educational strategy intended to change the beliefs, attitudes, values and structure of organisations so that they can better adapt to new technologies, markets and challenges, and the dizzying rate of change itself.

The final word on the true meaning of OD must go to Richard Beckhard, the doyen of OD and, in the view of many people, the man who did most to legitimise and in some sense even invent OD. During the 1990s I had the privilege of being taught by Richard Beckhard on two occasions in London, and they were two of those rare moments when you feel that you have been in touch with greatness. In his field he had become a 'legend in his lifetime', and the benefit of being taught by such a man will never leave me. At that time he must have been in his late eighties, and he had to sit in a chair for most of the day, but his mind was that of a young man, and the combination of learning and wisdom is something that one rarely encounters. At one event I witnessed him leading a master class where, through a one-to-one consulting session, he helped a chief executive of a large NHS trust to analyse her performance. It was awe-inspiring, in much the same way as watching a world-famous tenor instruct a novice and allowing music lovers to become voyeurs would be, and it put into practice Beckhard's observation that 'One purpose of OD is to help people be as effective as possible in the present, but another purpose is to prepare people for living in the different world of the future'.[5] And Beckhard's classic definition of OD remains the standard by which all others are judged:

OD is an effort planned, organisation-wide, and managed from the top, to increase organisation effectiveness and health through planned interventions in the organisation's 'processes', using behavioural-science knowledge.[6]

It is relatively easy to become pedantic and highlight the ways in which the academic-cum-practitioner definitions differ, but that seems to me to miss the point entirely. Of course there are variations in the words that are used, and of course there are emphases in different places to express the preferences of the writers, but the overriding fact that should strike a reader is the complementarity of their comments as they reflect on prism-like definitions from slightly different angles.

The variation in the very definition of OD revealed by these writers is also shown in the work of many practitioners and their preference for one type of OD intervention over another. In my work within healthcare I have been honoured to work with some wonderful people and their approaches to OD, and issues where they thought an OD intervention would be useful, have been diverse to say the least. The following five examples of different types of intervention, all taken from actual healthcare OD work in the UK, illustrate this point, and the examples are based on five composites of real people. No single example is based on just one individual, but despite this, and the fact that I have used fictitious names and changed some details, these former compatriots will no doubt recognise themselves, so I ask for understanding, and even forgiveness, if my caricatures offend.

KATH AND EMMA'S APPROACH

Kath, an NHS employee, is an academic to her fingertips. Throughout her career she has followed an evidence-based approach to most of her assignments, she has followed her seemingly natural instincts when it has come to developing research protocols and, as with most manager-academics, she sees adding to her list of publications, alongside the need to satisfy the demands of hospital management, as one of the major outcomes of any piece of work. Her approach is methodical – you can rely on the fact that she will have done a literature search on all of the relevant topics that are likely to arise and that there will be few things that she has not considered in advance.

Emma is a chartered occupational psychologist and is also employed by the NHS. She is younger than Kath, and eager to make a significant contribution to her chosen profession. She is a competent psychologist who knows the various applications that her work can bring to an assignment, but she is inexperienced in terms of applying that expertise to a practical healthcare management problem. Although a professional in her own right, she is likely to seek Kath's approval before she 'goes public' on a set of recommendations. She calls it the 'reality check' – she doesn't want to sound like a wet-behind-the-ears newly qualified graduate.

Kath and Emma had been commissioned to examine the level and causes of stress among medical consultants in a medium-sized general hospital. Their starting point was to examine whether or not a problem existed among the consultants, and to measure the extent of the problem. In order to obtain a relative measure they invited the consultants to participate in the study and sent each of them a questionnaire, suitably anonymised, designed to measure general aspects of healthy adjustment to stress. The questionnaire covered feelings of strain, depression, inability to cope, anxiety-based insomnia, lack of confidence and other psychological problems. Although the questionnaire was a self-report mechanism, and therefore would only record the subjective view of the person completing it, it had the advantage of being a nationally recognised method of gathering this type of information, with national norms available both for the general population and for this specific population group. A thorough statistical analysis of the returned questionnaires was undertaken, and the results were compared with those from a range of other studies using a similar approach. The study found substantially higher levels of stress than in similar groups of professional staff.

The second stage of the work set out to determine the causes of the stress using the Occupational Stress Indicator (OSI) to gather the quantitative data and a series of semi-structured interviews and discussion groups to gather the qualitative data. The causes were categorised under four headings, namely organisational forces, organisational structure and climate, managerial role and factors intrinsic to the job itself. Kath and Emma also made a set of recommendations and worked with the hospital management and consultants to introduce them. Everyone concerned believed that the assignment had been a success.

The work undertaken by Kath and Emma had been successful, but unfortunately it was not related to the fundamental and deep-lying real problems in this particular hospital. There were many other undeclared issues that needed to be addressed, and when they finally emerged many months later, they resulted in the hospital experiencing major problems. Kath and Emma cannot be blamed for this – they did what they were asked to do, they had no access to the wider hospital management agenda, and in their report to the executive directors they had pointed out that they were concerned that their work was doing little more than applying a solution – a 'sticking plaster' – to a symptom of something much more significant. The executive directors, probably for very good reasons at that stage, insisted on turning a blind eye to the wider and deeper issues.

My purpose is not to write a full account of Kath and Emma's work, or to diagnose the wider and deeper issues in this hospital, but to illustrate one approach to OD and how it addresses certain issues in an organisation. This approach was based on the application of behavioural science and an academic understanding of the literature for similar problems. The approach appealed to the scientific bent of the clients, it justified in their minds the rationale behind the set of recommendations, and it was the main reason for their acceptance and implementation of them.

ALISON'S APPROACH

Alison, another NHS employee, believed that hospitals should run like well-oiled machines – everything should be in its place, everything should be connected to something else by a set of organisational pulleys, and therefore OD meant intervening in the systems and processes of the hospital to ensure that all of its bits and pieces were pointing in the same direction and working to maximum effectiveness. Alison was a highly effective adviser and consultant, and her 'engineering' approach to OD was greatly valued by a wide range of hospital managers and clinicians.

A typical assignment for Alison would be to 'assure the Executive Team about the effectiveness of the existing roles, organisational arrangements and resource capacity/capability to deliver the Trust's agenda'. She loved it, and set about the task with the zeal of a railway enthusiast who has been asked to service a steam engine. She examined all of the internal and external 'key strategic documents', pored over 'organisational data such as minutes of corporate meetings, role profiles, objectives, staff attitude results, etc.', held 72 interviews with 'internal stakeholders', set up focus groups with a 'cross-section of managers and others', designed a diagnostic questionnaire 'to survey key players responsible for strategy implementation', and was not at all surprised when the response rate to her questionnaire was far in excess of a researcher's normal expectations.

One of the character-forming influences on her life had been Gary Hamel's view of 'several ways in which management processes are inimical to innovation'.[7] Among many other arguments, Hamel contends that most processes are calendar-driven and new opportunities can only arise within the structure of the planning round, that most management processes are biased towards conservation rather than growth, and that most management processes take the existing business model as the point of departure. Alison was determined that those charges would not be laid against any of her NHS colleagues/clients! The hospital processes, after she had finished with them, would be vibrant.

Her forensic skills knew no bounds, and she could boldly declare in the introduction to her set of recommendations:

> evidence has been gathered from a number of sources and therefore the project sponsors can be confident about the reliability of the emergent themes and the judgements made as a consequence. The team approach with regard to evidence gathering and analytical phases provides further assurances about the rigour and robustness of the findings.

When she asked the Trust board, whom she called the project sponsors (an interesting term in and of itself, and a choice of words that reflects her project management approach), to comment on 'the applicability and feasibility of the options put forward', it would be a brave or belligerent person who would question her well-researched and well-documented findings. I realise that my description of her methods makes her sound like a cold and analytical person, but nothing could be further from the truth – she was extremely pleasant company and charming to work alongside.

The point is that her method of applying OD within healthcare was focused on systems and procedures. Her report for this client identified a set of recommendations under the headings of culture, performance management, governance and risk management, management processes, corporate behaviour, structures, incentives/disincentives, customer involvement, capacity and capability, and development issues for individuals. Her report showed, with the help of a set of sensible diagrams and charts, how the whole thing should fit together and work effortlessly like a 'well-oiled machine'. She didn't add the last three words, but that is what she meant, and her use of phrases such as 'corporate machinery' symbolised the nature of her approach.

ADAM'S APPROACH

Adam is a 'people-person' and has worked in healthcare management all of his working life. He likes people and they like him. He engages in light-hearted banter with them and believes that harmony is a prerequisite of successful organisational life. That does not mean that he ducks those times when he has to act managerially and deal with an issue. In fact there are times when he can be quite tough, but he prefers to deal with issues from the perspective of understanding and developing relationships.

He is extremely skilled in understanding why people are behaving in a particular way – an understanding that has been developed further by his training in personality diagnostic techniques – and often he can achieve his goals by selecting the right time and method of intervention. He prevents misunderstandings from occurring by identifying the difficulties before most others do, and before they become an overt issue. He carries this view of the world into his OD work.

When Adam is presented with an OD assignment, the first thing he examines is the relationship issues within the hospital or community setting. He believes that almost any organisational structure can be made to work if the relationships are right, so for him the obvious first thing to look at is the harmony or lack of it between the senior people in the healthcare organisation and between them and the people they manage or lead. It is quite incredible to hear Adam recount a number of anecdotes about clinicians or managers who claimed to be a part of the same team but who allowed their natural antipathy for one another and their unhelpful competitive spirit to prevent the healthcare organisation from achieving what they both wanted it to achieve. Adam will unearth these problems and show the individuals concerned how the behavioural and relationship difficulties prevent them from realising their common goals. Sometimes he will use formal and less formal diagnostic instruments, but in most cases he will achieve his results by talking to people and, far more importantly, by getting them to talk honestly to one another by means of his expert facilitation. Adam is convinced that most people do not reveal how they feel about issues in their organisation, and often these hidden views are backed up by prejudices and deeply held beliefs about other people and departments that are just not true. Adam's ability to bring all of this out into the open and to work with clients to bring in new approaches to work and relationships is most productive and a boon to clients.

It would be rare for Adam to write a report with a set of recommendations – that would be far too formal. However, he will stay in touch with the client and make sure that he is on hand to work with them as further issues are identified. Inevitably there will be a need to act as a mentor or coach for the chief executive or clinical director, and that will have consequential effects for others in the hospital (or other setting), who will want to 'have their hand held' or 'access to an agony aunt', to use their expressions.

Adam has many OD facilitation interventions up his sleeve, and his favourite, when faced with two groups in a hospital who seem unable to get on with each other, is to place them in their natural work groupings and ask them to answer this question about the other group's perception of them: 'How do we think you see us?' It is hardly advanced science, yet it unearths long and deeply held beliefs about another group that are often completely untrue or a distortion of the facts. Most of Adam's interventions are, on the face of it, quite innocuous, yet they are based on his confidence with people, his vast experience and his belief that ironing out relationship problems can have a dramatic effect on a healthcare organisation's overall performance.

Adam's style is not unique. The writer Colin Carnall[8] identifies blockages to effective change under five helpful headings:

1 perceptual blocks, such as stereotyping
2 emotional blocks, such as the fear of making a mistake
3 cultural blocks, such as taboos – issues that cannot be discussed
4 environmental blocks, such as not accepting criticism
5 cognitive blocks, such as the incorrect use of language.

Adam is the personification of the blockbuster. Whether they are perceptual, emotional, cultural, environmental or cognitive blocks, you can rely on Adam to help you to overcome them.

PETER'S APPROACH

Peter trained as a microbiologist and then worked as a schoolteacher. This initial discipline influenced his understanding and application of OD when he joined the world of healthcare management – he saw OD as needing to be interpreted through a whole-system view of the world. He is one of the few people I have worked with who truly understood and could debate in immense detail Senge's influential systems-based masterpiece, *The Fifth Discipline*.[9] He could grasp the intricacies of that text and could even appreciate, in a manner where real meaning and learning occurred, the scientific view of organisations taken by writers such as Margaret Wheatley.[10] Peter would develop computer-based systems that would map the full extent of the issues that his primary care colleagues/clients had rather naively and short-sightedly thought only pertained to one part of the healthcare system. He was able to demonstrate to an awe-struck GP that the issues described were part of a much greater whole and that a solution could only be reached if an integrated 'whole-system' view was taken. The GP could even be heard to mutter about the systemic nature of his challenges! Practice after practice came to appreciate Peter and saw him as an extremely valuable colleague.

Peter really enjoyed drawing diagrams, but these diagrams (drawn with the assistance of a computer package, of course) were like no other diagrams you have ever seen. They resembled the electronic circuitry of a space rocket – they were so elaborate yet, with some explanation from Peter, they made perfect sense to the clinicians and service users. What is more, when Peter had placed them on a wall, with the help of vast quantities of Blu-Tack and Post-it labels, he would invite to a meeting/workshop every person who made a contribution to the system he had just mapped. It was astonishing to witness a crowd of people examining his system map in detail and identifying the location of their glorious effort on behalf of the organisation, or from their position as clinician or patient. The most extraordinary discovery in the whole process was made when the main players in the system – doctors, nurses, social workers, hospital consultants, managers and also patients – came to realise that they had not previously understood how the overall system worked and how their actions impinged upon the work of others and, most importantly, on the overall performance of the service and the experience of patients. Their responses were sometimes exhilarating as they worked collaboratively to suggest ways in which the local healthcare system could be improved. Each suggestion led to changes being made to the 'wiring diagram' and a debate on the likely consequences of such a set of actions.

Overall, the whole-system view that Peter gave them led to measurable improvements in the care given and created a sense of involvement among the key players. There was also a greater sense of the 'domino effect' of their decisions on other parts of the healthcare system, and Peter would sometimes be hailed as a mini-miracle worker by clients who would not accept his protestations that all he had done was to draw a picture, or a map, of what they had told him.

WALT'S APPROACH

This is the fifth and final approach, and I have left it to last became I am not particularly sympathetic with Walt's approach. Walt refers to what he calls *organisational development*, and in my experience the use of the suffix '-al' at the end of the word is often (but not always) a signal that the person using the term believes that OD is a more sophisticated term and a grander way of reorganising and restructuring the hospital. That is Walt's belief. When he talks about *organisational development*, you can be pretty sure that in a moment or two a set of newly drawn organisational charts – he sometimes calls them organigrams – will be revealed. He looks at them admiringly, and sincerely believes that the answers to the latest round of problems and challenges can all be met by reorganising the hospital. He agrees wholeheartedly when it is pointed out to him that changing the organisation structure is often the easiest part of a change strategy, and that the real work, still to be addressed by Walt, concerns attitudinal and behavioural change. He records the need for these issues to be tackled – what he considers to be the softer end of the OD intervention – on his flipchart, but you know and he knows that they are most unlikely to be tackled. The emphasis will be on changing the structures, more and more reorganisation, more and more disruption to the smooth running of the hospital, and less and less treatment of those soft but oh-so-important behavioural issues.

He obviously has not realised the truth identified by Rosabeth Moss Kanter,[11] who shows that 'restructurings can provide a long catalogue of threats to value retention' in an organisation. She identifies the main items as the costs of confusion, misinformation, emotional leakage, loss of energy, loss of key resources, breakdown of initiative and a weakened faith in leaders' ability.

There are times when Walt is absolutely right, and the greatest need of the hospital is to have a change in its structures. It may be too centralised as an organisation to achieve its aims, or there may be an imbalance between clinical and supporting service areas. Walt sees these occasional needs for structural change as a vindication of his entire approach to each and every OD problem: 'if something is not working as effectively as it ought to be working, there is a need to change the organisation's structures' is his entire approach to life. This apparent vindication blinds him to the times when changing the structures has had little effect, or even a negative effect, on the situation. When it is crystal clear to everyone that the latest reorganisation has been less than a glowing success, Walt is adept at explaining that this problem has been caused by an unforeseen change in circumstances or by the inexperience or lack of expertise of those given the task of implementing his grand design.

BRINGING THE FIVE APPROACHES TOGETHER

Before I introduced these six people and five approaches to OD, I emphasised that they were caricatures although they are based on a composite of real people in the world of healthcare. With the exception of Walt's predilection for changing the structure of hospitals and for reorganising anything that stands still for too long, I have over-emphasised Kath and Emma's use of behavioural science, Alison's diagnosis of processes and systems, Adam's reliance on people skills and Peter's belief in mapping whole systems, in order to make a very significant point. All of the approaches are valid, even Walt's, but there can be a danger when an OD expert becomes too wedded to just one approach at the expense of others. Most successful OD practitioners understand the need for a diversity of approaches (as the first five names in my examples do in real life), and that using a mixture of approaches for a range of different circumstances is extremely important.

This practical example of different people approaching OD challenges in different ways also highlights the richness inherent in the many definitions of OD. These definitions are not contradictory but complementary, and they reflect the breadth of activity that comes under the banner of OD. The written definitions, plus the practical examples, should reinforce the point that OD covers a multitude of approaches and that a truly skilled practitioner can help a healthcare executive or clinician to unlock the full potential within an organisation. And as I show later, most of these OD skills can be practised by healthcare staff without the need for recourse to expensive external management consultants.

Different conceptual frameworks abound, and although there can be a danger in an OD person appearing to be slavishly bound to one framework over another, one would expect someone who claimed to be an expert on organisation development to have assimilated the various models into their practice, in much the same way as a driver has absorbed the Highway Code into the way they drive. The most popular frameworks are: Marvin Weisbord's six-box model,[12] a diagnostic framework published in 1976, which uses six critical areas; the 7S model popularised by Peters and Waterman;[13] Senge's[14] work on organisational learning; planned change models[15] (Lewin's unfreezing-movement-freezing change model and the action research model are examples); and others use initiatives such as the European Foundation for Quality Management and the Balanced Scorecard techniques as a successful surrogate or partner for an OD programme.

Later in this chapter I shall outline the Richard Beckhard model favoured by many.

MANAGING CHANGE

Most efforts at change fall short of their goals. As Peter Senge and his colleagues report, many of their efforts to create learning organisations did not accomplish the intended results. Ron Ashkenas writes that only 25 to 30 per cent of change efforts actually succeed. James Champy shares similar findings about his work on re-engineering, reporting success rates of about 25 to 33 per cent. Clearly, interventions – no matter how well intentioned and carefully thought out – are far more difficult to put into action than we think.[16]

Why is managing change so difficult? Why does it cause fear and alarm in so many people? Why do some people violently oppose change?

Academics from the Massachusetts Institute of Technology (MIT),[17] through their work on organisational learning, believe that there are 10 specific objections and challenges that have to be dealt with before there is any chance of managing change successfully. They are attitudes typified by comments such as these: 'We don't have time for this stuff!', 'We have no help!', 'This stuff isn't relevant!', 'We have the right way! They don't understand us!' A range of other similar and well-worn phrases that reveal a fundamental disquiet with proposed change are known by everyone who has attempted to introduce change.

MIT's 10 reasons are reinforced by the writings of Dave Ulrich,[18] a man who has done more than most to demonstrate the credibility of human resource management and its direct link to the performance of the organisation. He also identified 10 reasons (in note form) to explain why he believes 'changes don't produce change'. These included not being tied to strategy, grandiose expectations versus simple successes, lack of leadership about changes, and being unable to mobilise commitment to sustain change.

These lists substantiate the experience of people in many healthcare organisations, but they also represent an indictment of the way in which far too many organisations set about introducing change. Can you imagine a healthcare or any other organisation introducing change that is not connected to strategy? Are there healthcare organisations out there using change as a fad or as a 'quick-fix' (I ask somewhat disingenuously!)? Are they employing short-term perspectives and then wondering why there is a lack of tangible results? And are they engaging in change initiatives because they are merely 'reinventing the wheel' or because their leaders are not 'walking the talk'? Unfortunately, the answer is sometimes in the affirmative.

Practising change

As I practised change management over the years, occasionally in some extremely hostile environments, I always held the view that there were some elementary steps that could be taken to make change happen more effectively. In later years, as I studied change management – yes, I confess, I practised it before studying it! – I came to see that despite the numerous tomes written on the subject, there is usually an elementary set of steps at the heart of all sensible change management messages. There are three seminal works (or to be more accurate, two seminal books and one bravura conference performance) that have influenced my thinking on change.

The first book is a masterpiece. Written by Richard Beckhard and Reuben Harris, *Organizational Transitions*[19] is a classic, and one of those rare books where every page contains a combination of academic rigour and practical management relevance. Any leader involved in the challenge of change should avail themselves of a copy of this text and luxuriate in the fact that each of Beckhard and Harris's steps resonates with the experience of healthcare managers – the simply described, yet wise and effective techniques have been proven to work time and time again. In Stage 1 there is a need to examine the options for change and to explain to the people involved the limited range of options. In Stage 2 it is essential to 'describe the future state' (how often have organisations plunged in without a clear sense of where they are heading?). In Stage 4 there is a need for a clear transition plan. I could go on, but any summary of their book does not do it justice. It is a masterpiece, and should be required reading for any manager engaged in change.

The second book is also essential reading. It contains John Kotter's *eight steps for successful large-scale change*,[20] and in it he argues for a systematic approach to bringing about successful change. His well-publicised eight steps include building the guiding team and making change stick.

When I gave a copy of Kotter's book to a colleague who is a chief executive of a large NHS trust, he was not impressed. I gave it to him for the simple reason that he was concerned with the way in which change was being handled in his trust and I, rather tactfully I thought, believed that starting a change process in the way Kotter proposed might be helpful to the organisation. He dismissed the book as being 'too much like a basic formula for change and no more than a "Highway Code" approach'. My colleague intended his words as a criticism of the book, whereas I saw them as a compliment. Kotter's book, based on his extensive research, is far more than a simple formula or a Highway Code, but even at the level of a Highway Code the book's messages are crucially important and, as with a Highway Code, the key principles need to become absorbed into one's psyche and then practised subliminally.

The third seminal work was a conference speech delivered by Rosabeth Moss Kanter in Cardiff in 1993.[21] It was superb, and for over an hour I sat listening to this intellectual colossus among management thinkers explain her views on managing change. She dominated the stage and, without the benefit of any visible notes and without visual aids, she held her large audience in the palm of her hand. She told us (and here I rely on the rather scribbled notes that I took at the time) that in order to implement change effectively leaders must ensure that they have:

1 lined up the key stakeholders behind them
2 a clear vision that is shared by their associates
3 ensured that there is active and energetic communication of the vision and that it is translated into concrete steps for everyone
4 a clear management guidance system to co-ordinate matters

5 plenty of room left for local experiment; local departments must do it in their own way – they should experiment
6 found out what is getting in the way of implementing the vision (e.g. information systems, rewards, people)
7 standards and measures to assess successes
8 sent signals and created symbols of the new heroes.

It was a magnificent speech, although one is left wondering how many of her principles and words of wisdom were put into practice by those who experienced the orgasmic feeling of hearing Kanter in full flow. Later that week, or it may have been on one of her later visits to the UK, I was privileged to be part of a private dinner function at the King's Fund where she spoke quite informally. Again she was heard by the 20 or so healthcare staff with rapt attention as she explained her thinking on an aspect of leadership. A truly impressive person and performance.

Practical points about change

Before leaving the subject of change I want to share some of the practical points that many healthcare clients have found to be helpful in their challenge to bring about effective change.

1 Do not become over-reliant on a stated theory or theoretical approach. It is dangerous to be wedded to a single approach and to be unable to move with the flow of events or to take hold of an unexpected opportunity. It would be a tragedy to miss a golden opportunity to take things forward because you happen to be at Stage 3 of your change agenda and this opportunity should not, in theory, be discussed until Stage 7 or 8. Anyone with experience will know that there are times when it is necessary to take what is being presented, to make the most of it and be grateful for it, and then to improvise the next stages after the opportunity has been grasped. As I facilitated one challenging change programme, I was asked by a public health consultant 'What you suggest works in practice, but does it work in theory?' He was half-joking, I'm sure, but there is more than a grain of truth in what he said, and it should ring alarm bells for managers and internal facilitators. To be aware of the dangers of over-reliance on the theoretical approach and to use an understanding of theory to make practice highly effective should be everyone's guiding principle.

2 Beware of what many academics and commentators call the *Heathrow School of Management*. This term refers to the type of book that can be bought as one waits to board a plane. It usually contains an overly simple description of how it is possible to overcome every imaginable challenge and succeed in the world of management. Life is far more complex than these books suggest, and plunging into some complicated campaign on the basis of their advice can be extremely dangerous. Before I leave this point, I should say that the term *Heathrow School of Management* applies to a certain type of book, and not to Heathrow *per se*. I know from personal experience that Heathrow airport sells a range of excellent books, as well as those with a somewhat lesser pedigree.

3   Some people are tempted to deal with the challenge of change as they would deal with an objective or quasi-scientific problem, where they believe that they understand all of the issues and that they have these variables under control. It is wise to recognise that some of the variables are often beyond one's control, especially those unexpected issues that invariably crawl out from underneath someone or something and proceed to bite you. The wise and experienced manager or clinician, or internal change agent, will have a set of a contingency plans, but despite these plans there will inevitably be an unexpected issue, and even with the benefit of hindsight it will be an issue that would have been difficult to spot.

4   Beware of the autocratic and belligerent type of manager, fortunately a rare breed in healthcare, who believes that he or she can introduce change by a word of command and expects the change to make a fundamental difference to the organisation in the long term. I was once asked to work with the chief executive of a well-known UK organisation (not in healthcare, I emphasise), whose attitude to change was summed up in one of his favourite phrases: 'When they hear the sound of my jackboots coming down the corridor they'll change'. He was right – in the short term, people did change and outwardly they did conform to his requirements, but they held a substantial resentment about his management style, and after a relatively short time many of the ablest people in the organisation left to take up other, more attractive, posts. It was such a shame, as the organisation needed top-class people because it faced huge challenges, but the attitude of the chief executive drove them out, and although I feel that my interventions ameliorated some of the worst excesses, they were insufficient to change the personality of a man who wanted to dominate his organisation. What is surprising is that he never found it difficult to recruit high-quality replacements for the staff who had left. There was a belief in this organisation, and the sector it occupied, that if you could work for a right b****** like X for two years it did your credibility a lot of good. Unfortunately, chief executive X never figured out the reason for his recruitment successes. I have also come across variations of this behaviour in other sectors, including healthcare, where managers, often at much lower levels than chief executive, believed a hard, tough management approach to change to be the most productive one and summed up their management philosophy with the phrase 'If you grab them by the b**** then their hearts and minds will follow'.

5   It is useful to reflect on the type of change that has to be managed. The diagram in Figure 2.1, taken from an NHS publication,[22] is extremely useful and helps the client to muse on the difference between change that is in reality little more than an extrapolation of the past practices, change that is a paradigm shift where there is a need to produce a new way of operating, and cataclysmic change that is needed to prevent the organisation from 'going out of business'. This simple device is usually highly productive, as it helps the client to think about the nature of the change, the different strategies that can be employed, and the costs of success, failure and partial implementation. With the appropriate facilitation, the diagram will often help the client to construct an action plan and a 'balance sheet' of the costs and benefits of change.

6 There are times when the client will agree wholeheartedly with the proposition that there is a need to 'define the future state', but will have genuine difficulty in doing so as they will be able to identify a number of imponderables. When this happens, which is quite often, the diagram shown in a book on management strategy[23] is extremely helpful, as it demonstrates to the client that it is quite usual to have the degree of uncertainty they are experiencing (you can almost hear the sigh of relief) and that it is sensible to map out two or even three potential future states and to engage in some contingency or scenario planning in which all of the eventualities are covered.

7 The following are the six points of advice that I find myself giving most often to healthcare colleagues who are facing change.

- It is essential to have a clear idea of the future state or states that you wish to achieve. It is very clear that if you do not know where you are going you will not know when you have got there, and it will be nigh impossible to convince your workforce that the change is being led by a credible management.

- It takes large amounts of energy and perseverance to see through a change programme, and there is a danger that the person who visualised and articulated the change will become bored by the implementation stages and will seek new visions and ideas. Someone must drive through the implementation phases.

- As you concentrate on the changes that you want to introduce, it is easy to take your eye off the current agenda and to miss problems as they arise, or even new service opportunities. Managing the present while creating the future is essential.

- Some managers will look to outsiders to provide them with advice. Some of this consultancy advice may be substandard, so it is essential that external advisers are chosen very carefully.

- It is nigh on impossible to communicate sufficiently. Choose every method, and still be concerned that insufficient attention has been paid to the matter. When you have communicated via every possible channel, do not become angry when someone who should know better says to you that they did not know, or did not realise, that such and such was about to happen.

- Celebrate even small successes, and go out of your way to reward changed behaviour – the behaviour that your change programme is trying to achieve.

One famous management guru and writer has a wonderful illustration to highlight the way in which leaders can no longer rely on:

> the old rules of traditional, hierarchical, high-external-control, top-down management . . . [and so need to create] . . . a sense of vision that people are drawn to . . . that enables them to be driven by inner motivation toward achieving a common purpose.[24]

He asks the people he is working with, and these are usually large audiences, to

Developmental change
Improvement of existing situation

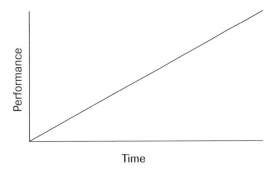

...nsitional change
Implementation of a known new state:
management of the interim transition
state over a controlled period of time

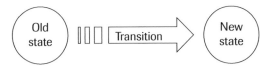

Transformational change
Emergence of a new state, unknown
until it takes shape out of the remains
of the chaotic death of the old state;
time period not easily controlled

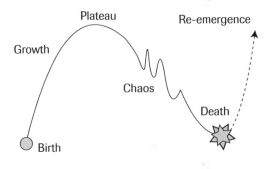

FIGURE 2.1 Perspectives on change
Source: Iles V and Sutherland K (2001) *Managing Change in the NHS:*
organisational change. Department of Health, London.

close their eyes and point in the direction of north. He then asks them to open
their eyes and see where everyone is pointing. Without exception, people are
pointing in just about every possible direction. When I've used this illustration
I've even had people pointing at the ceiling because, as they explain to me later,
they thought I wanted them to 'understand that north is up there somewhere'.
The guru then asks only those who are certain of the direction of north to repeat
the exercise. The outcome is very similar, and he uses this powerful illustration
to demonstrate the difficulty of setting a direction for the employees of an
organisation in a dynamic, ever-changing world.

It is an illustration that travels well across the Atlantic, and it becomes a
sound launching pad to reinforce a message that most people in healthcare
organisations already know, namely that to be a successful leader in today's
world of complex organisations often requires new skills and new approaches.

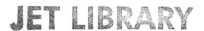

The old-style command and control system of management possesses a dinosaur-like quality, and all too often it no longer works in a world occupied by a younger generation of employees, especially where the ascendancy of the independent-minded knowledge worker is taking place. However, knowing that there is a need to bring about a fundamental change in the style of management is one thing, but translating this into effective practice is something else.

I have worked with some senior teams who, convinced of the need to set a clear direction for the organisation and to prepare a statement of values that allows a highly decentralised and quasi-autonomous professional staff to follow this overall direction, appear to believe that the mere act of agreeing and issuing the statements is the entire management task. They seem to believe that the statements will mysteriously transfer themselves, almost by a process of organisational osmosis, into the minds, hearts and actions of hundreds, maybe even thousands of their staff. Obviously they believe in miracles. After a short while they are astonished to discover that their carefully crafted, impressive statements are not being followed, and even the most loyal of staff have difficulty remembering whether they ever received a copy of the values statement.

CASE STUDY 2.1

In one public-sector organisation where I worked in an advisory capacity, the chief executive was extremely proud of his statement of purpose and set of principles. They had been laboured over by the Chief Executive Officer (CEO) and the senior management team. In fairness, they were impressive – beautifully crafted – and the CEO had been careful to include them in various corporate and operational plans that set out the direction for the next five years. In fact, the senior management team was so proud of them that it made the grave mistake of inviting the chairman, the CEO's boss, to a review meeting that the team was holding with the organisation's other senior managers. What became clear very quickly, and to the horror of the CEO, was that the remaining senior managers of the organisation knew very little about the scope and significance of the statement of purpose and set of principles. Many of them could remember receiving a copy, but some could not. Many knew that they represented a significant document for the organisation, but others did not. Some had been told about them in their regular team briefing session, but others quite clearly did not have regular team briefings. The CEO was horrified, but experience prevailed and he expertly overcame a potentially embarrassing event. His chairman, a very experienced and highly respected individual, understood perfectly what had happened and was also wise enough to understand why it had happened.

That afternoon, chastened by his experience, the CEO sent his senior staff an email that politely but firmly reminded them that the statement of purpose and set of principles had been circulated to them many weeks ago both by email and in traditional paper format, and had been included in the various corporate and operational plans, if they cared to look at these. Although his email was fairly temperate, it was obvious that he was livid with his staff for letting him down in front of the chairman. The chairman saw it as an opportunity for a coaching session between him and the CEO.

CASE STUDY 2.2

On another occasion, I remember sitting around the board table of a healthcare organisation with an executive group, of which I was one of the directors. We were discussing the main initiatives being implemented as part of the quality management programme. Forty minutes into the meeting we realised that the CEO, who was chairing the meeting, had a different list of initiatives from the one in front of the rest of the executives! For the first 30 minutes of the meeting this had made little difference, as most of the executives were clearly 'going through the motions' and their minds were not properly engaged. The CEO's list had 48 initiatives and ours had a mere 34. Can you believe that this organisation had over 80 quality initiatives on the go at the same time? To the credit of the CEO, he laughed when the discrepancy was pointed out to him, and all of the directors learned from the experience and applied the very significant lesson in future meetings.

Case studies 2.1 and 2.2 are classic examples of the 'true-north principle'. It is one thing to know that north is up and south is down, and that west is to the left of east when you look at a compass, but it is quite another thing to be able to point in the direction of north when someone asks you to do it in an unfamiliar environment. And it is exactly the same with mission and value statements or any other healthcare management strategy. Drawing them up is the easy part. The real challenge lies in inculcating them into the minds and hearts of the staff of the organisation so that their actions, consciously and even subliminally, conform to the values, the mission and the strategies that have been set out. It is not that employees should become automatons – that is the last thing that is wanted – but it means that as a result of the investment made in communicating the direction and values of the organisation, colleagues act in a way that is consistent with what the strategies are trying to achieve. The phrase 'winning the hearts and minds of your people' has become an overworked cliché, but it remains an important principle and one that is extremely difficult to achieve.

All healthcare organisations need people who are internal change agents. Occasionally, there is a need for experts to be brought in from outside the organisation, but usually there are people within the healthcare organisation who have developed their own expertise as internal change agents.

The eight facilitator roles

In my experience there are eight different ways in which clients at different levels of a typical healthcare organisation make use of a facilitator. This says a great deal about individual managers and their organisation, and is a source of constant amusement for the facilitator – 'How will they try to use me today?' is a constant thought. The eight facilitator types are presented in no particular order of frequency, significance or importance. The different approaches are offered to help managers and clinicians to decide how they can best help their organisation by becoming an internal facilitator or, at the very least, by becoming more facilitative in their management style.

1 Surrogate manager

A golden rule for any facilitator is that they should never cross the line between facilitator and client and carry out the job of managing in the place of the client. The facilitator is happy to help in the construction of an appropriate strategy, to analyse and comment on certain management practices, and to work with the client to develop an action plan. However, the facilitator should never perform the management job for the client. Undertaking the role of an interim or locum manager is quite another issue. Yet there are times when the 'client' is keen for the facilitator to cross the line and adopt a managerial style of intervention. The client may be happy to take the back seat and allow the facilitator to drive the organisation forward on a particular issue, and it has often puzzled me why this should be the case. I think there are two principal reasons.

First, the client may be a mediocre manager and therefore be only too happy for someone else to take the required action. Or it may be that the manager recognises that the facilitator has a better management track record, or that the expertise of the facilitator is far more relevant on this occasion. Usually this is a deserved expertise, although occasionally the facilitator's expertise may be enhanced merely by the fact that they are the person from outside the immediate organisation – we all know that 'prophets in their own country' often have a difficult time convincing people of the relevance of their knowledge and expertise.

The second principal reason for encouraging the facilitator to act as manager is far more Machiavellian. The manager is happy for the facilitator to take the lead as it gives the manager a 'second bite of the cherry' if amendments are needed, such as the action plan or the draft strategy not quite hitting the mark. This is the opportunity the Machiavellian has been waiting for. With perfect timing, the manager makes the necessary amendments and demonstrates, in one bold move and with consummate skill, what they believe to be improvements in the work undertaken by the facilitator, who did not quite understand the finer points of the issues. The manager is a hero, or at least this is what they believe when they look in the mirror. Their bosses may know better.

2 Priest

Being a boss can be a lonely experience. The higher one rises in an organisation, the fewer people there are with whom to share one's problems and inner thoughts. One of the roles of the facilitator is that of 'priest', and as the facilitator and client develop their relationship they will often jokingly refer to some coaching sessions as times in the 'confessional box'. For many senior people a problem shared really is a problem halved, and the therapeutic quality of getting something 'off one's chest' or 'speaking out loud one's thoughts' and then receiving a response from someone with expertise and a truly independent and impartial view should not be underestimated. Although it is harder for an internal facilitator to demonstrate independence and impartiality, it is not impossible, and of course the insider's difficulty in this area is more than compensated for by the fact that they have a better grasp of the full extent of the issues.

Take the example of Phil (not his real name). He was the chief executive of a large healthcare organisation employing thousands of staff that, to all intents and purposes, and certainly in the estimation of the outside world, was very successful. Phil had a series of interconnecting problems to deal with. His relationships with the board were not what they should have been, and he was being challenged on some key strategic items. Two of his senior directors were at loggerheads with each other and both were doing their utmost to undermine the other's performance. Yet another of his senior directors was suspected of practice likely to cause audit problems, even if proof was difficult to find. There was a personality clash between Phil and one of his major stakeholders, and in addition to all of this his wife was unwell. (All of these facts are taken from a real-life case, somewhere in the UK, although I have written them in a way that disguises Phil's real identity.)

As far as people could tell everything in the healthcare organisation was fine, but inside the organisation it was a very different story. When Phil came to meet me, he chose the venue carefully, and the conversation went something like this:

Phil: 'Hi Stephen. Can I tell you briefly what the issues are?'

Me: 'Sure. Would you like some coffee?'

Phil: 'No thanks, I've just had one. It's like this.'

And for the next 63 minutes, with the occasional nod or smile of understanding from me, Phil told me his problems. It was obviously a cathartic experience for him and it was quite evident that the relief was palpable. For the first time in weeks, and perhaps even months, he was not the only person who knew the full extent of these serious problems. We talked for another hour and I made some suggestions, but I am not sure that he was really listening to me as his mind was consumed with the challenges that he faced. That was the last time I saw him, because shortly afterwards he decided to resign his post.

Inevitably, I wonder whether there was more that I could have done. Should I have contacted him at home? At the time it seemed to be wisest to give him time and space. No one expected him to resign, and I am not sure that further sessions with a facilitator would have rescued the dire set of circumstances with which he had to cope. Yet this experience, as well as countless others, convinces me of the legitimacy of the facilitator undertaking the role of organisational priest. Absolution may not be possible, but having someone to talk to and being given sensible advice are invaluable.

An internal facilitator might think, with some justification, that it would have been impossible to talk to one's own chief executive about such personal and sensitive issues. That is probably true, but what this case illustrated was the fact that an internal facilitator would have had numerous opportunities to intervene before many of the issues cumulatively became too much for Phil to handle. Many of the issues could have been 'nipped in the bud' and, who knows, perhaps there might have been a very different outcome.

3 *Doctor*

In this relationship, the client will explain in some detail the healthcare organisation's problems (perhaps the words *ailments* or *pains* reflect the metaphor of doctor more accurately) and then – although the client is not naive enough to ask for the equivalent of two pills to take at mealtimes, or the ointment to rub in twice a day – there is an expectation that the facilitator will produce the perfect remedy.

For a minority of clients, the ideal remedy would be one that worked instantaneously, would not require surgery of any kind, and would result in the patient feeling almost superhuman once more. Other more mature clients realise that they will have to take 'tablets' or rub in a 'lotion' for a number of weeks before the problems will be eased, but even more mature clients realise that on the whole there are no quick fixes to most problems, and that the work of the facilitator will be effective over a longer period of time. The mature client appreciates the best use of the facilitator – in doctor mode the facilitator will act as a diagnostician, work with the client to examine the problems of the organisation and its people and, over time, produce a remedy or solution.

This is a legitimate role, and the metaphor carries with it an apt description of the activities designed to smooth out an organisation's troubles. It is an especially relevant metaphor in the world of healthcare. However, implicit in this metaphor is the fact that the facilitator, like all good doctors, should always undertake diagnostic work before recommending a prescription. Yet this approach does not always please the client, who may have a pet theory on the best way to tackle a particular problem. There are even some external facilitators, under commercial pressure to sell a new concept, who will be tempted to sell a partially tried and tested solution from the metaphorical 'bottle on the shelf'. Whatever the reason and no matter how strong the temptation, the internal facilitator should always regard the principle of diagnosis preceding prescription as sacrosanct.

4 *Boffin*

Closely related to the role of doctor is that of boffin. The facilitator may be seen as the expert in the field – rightly so in many instances – and because the client has such an issue to deal with there is an expectation that a contribution from this boffin is all that is required. There are occasions when this is true, and many specialist areas come to mind. In cases where there is a clear-cut speciality the contribution of an expert should be listened to and implemented. Indeed, not to do this would be bad practice.

In other cases the issue of expertise is not so clear-cut. In these circumstances the facilitator has to be careful to distinguish between incontrovertible fact, evidence-based research that may be open to challenge, best practice in other healthcare organisations, and those things that it is for the client to decide upon and implement. So long as the client clearly understands the various qualifications placed on advice given, playing the part of the boffin can be a useful facilitation role.

There are some organisations that act without recourse to the welter of research, management books, case studies and even the precedents that exist within their own organisations. It is quite astonishing to observe the extent to which the 'left hand' and the 'right hand' within an organisation do not know the lessons learned by their own colleagues on similar matters. What a glorious opportunity this presents for the aspiring internal facilitator. He or she ought to draw upon these various sources of intelligence and help the client to make better-informed decisions. Those managers in the organisation who have a need to understand the theory underpinning some course of action will praise such interventions, whereas without such evidence they may view the actions of their chief executive as somewhat gung-ho.

5 Engineer

The well-running machine needs some oiling. Alternatively, there may be a breakdown that needs to be repaired. Both of these examples fit the metaphor of engineer, but the cardinal point of this metaphor is that the client wants the facilitator to get his or her hands dirty – covered in oil – in order to prove that the facilitator belongs to the real world and is not just some theory-based type.

Most organisations have some form of initiation rite. In the 1960s, when heavy industry was at its height, there were rituals concerned with weights and toxic fumes. In the health service such rites may be concerned with a visit to some part of the pathology department. In some parts of the public sector they can involve the volume of work that someone is able to handle before stress kicks in, or they may involve attendance at a difficult board meeting with a chairman who can make the toughest manager tremble. Initiation is one of the ritualistic processes that feature in most cultures.

Once the facilitator has shown an ability to cope with these challenges there is often proper engineering work to be done. Well-running machines need to be oiled and broken-down engines have to be repaired.

The principle is clear for both the external and internal facilitator. It is essential for the facilitator to demonstrate the ability to deliver the goods in the toughest of internal environments. To change the metaphor somewhat, the facilitator has to show the capacity to stand in the trenches alongside the senior manager with the ability to 'slug it out' should a battle arise.

6 Ambassador

This role is often expected of the facilitator by managers at levels below those at which the facilitator normally operates. They know that the facilitator works at director and chief executive level, and for them those are the corridors of power. It may be that the facilitator represents their only actual contact with the upper echelons of management and, no matter how tenuous the connection, they intend to make the most of the opportunity.

They see the facilitator as an ambassador, someone who may have influence at board level – the court of the organisation's rulers – and they would like to be represented by the facilitator as a manager who does a first-class job. They think that the facilitator might commend their work for the organisation in a conversation with a director or the chief executive. So the middle managers set out to impress the facilitator with their achievements and their management style. Loyalty to the cause is also expressed, and they usually want to prove this by disclosing that they work long hours. As facilitators should operate under a strict code of conduct that demands client confidentiality, the efforts of the middle managers are usually wasted. The facilitator, even if impressed by the contributions of these managers, is hardly likely to disclose anything about them to a client, or to the chief executive, in another part of the healthcare organisation.

Sometimes there is a variation in the approach of the middle managers, as they see the facilitator as someone who can influence the bosses on an issue of organisational policy. Their interest is not primarily focused on the advancement of their own career, but on the development of some concept within the organisation. They see the facilitator as an influential yet neutral contributor to the policy-making process. At other times the reverse is true and they see the facilitator as a representative of senior management, and an unpopular policy. Although they understand that the facilitator is not a part of the senior management team, nevertheless this is their opportunity to express hostility to someone who is associated, however remotely, with the senior management of the organisation. They reveal their opposition to full effect, and the experienced facilitator will know that there are times when it is necessary to stand there, allow the angst to be expressed, allow them to vent their spleen and antagonism towards the organisation, treat their comments seriously, and ask their permission to report these comments to senior management on an anonymous basis. There are times when this has to be done before there is any chance of moving the agenda forward.

7 Fall guy

A problem arises and action has to be taken to resolve it. The manager's boss has to be convinced that the manager is being proactive and doing something to address the issues. What can be done? The answer – call in a facilitator.

Most of the time this is a perfectly fair arrangement, and over time the problems can be solved with the help of a facilitator. However, there are times when the facilitator is being used as a decoy. First of all it buys time for the manager – the boss can be told that action is being taken to resolve the problem. Secondly, the manager hopes that either something will turn up to change the circumstances which gave rise to the problem – the age-old strategy whereby if you do nothing about a problem for long enough it might just go away – or difficulties elsewhere will reduce the pressure that is being exerted by the boss.

Thirdly, the manager can try to use the facilitator as a fall guy. This is done by commissioning a piece of work from the facilitator and then undermining the work by attempting to change the terms of reference during the period of facilitation and/or by delaying implementation of the action plan under some spurious pretext. The facilitator, unless he or she is experienced in these dark arts and adept at avoiding them, can be trapped and suffer a tarnished reputation as a result. The manager can blame the lack of progress on the fact that the facilitator did not 'deliver the goods', and a busy boss can be placated by this for a time.

8 Audience member

Some managers are entertainers. Give them an audience and they will stand up and perform 20 minutes of their act. 'Act' is not a pejorative word in this context, as they can be thoroughly entertaining. They love an audience, even if it consists of just one facilitator, and they can keep themselves entertained for hours by telling of their latest strategic initiatives. Anyone who has seen the BBC TV series *The Office* will know only too well how David Brent treated his trainer/facilitator and eventually forced him to leave the assignment.

Chris is such a manager. You just have to watch his eyes dancing around, his arms waving about, his sudden movement to the enormous whiteboard opposite his desk, the speed with which ideas are introduced, arrows are drawn, and three overlapping circles are produced. He is entertaining, a joy to be with and, in fairness to him, he will listen and process other people's ideas into his view of the world and his list of key priorities. As a member of his audience it is important to go with the flow, a current being generated by the dynamism of his personality.

Caroline also loves an audience. She will tell you ad nauseam about her achievements and the ways in which she is tackling various issues. She will produce file after file, case studies, personal recollections, and lists of her well-connected colleagues, and her stamina will appear to be inexhaustible. The one difference is that she is not interested in listening to the views of a mere facilitator. For her the adrenalin rush comes from telling of her heroic deeds, and where there is evidence that another approach may have resulted in better dividends it is something that, no matter how delicately phrased, falls on deaf ears. She needs outside help, but will only find it in moments of deepest crisis.

Working with Chris is fun. Working with Caroline is nigh on impossible.

So there you have it – eight different roles that the facilitator is called upon to play. The majority are legitimate roles, but some of them should be treated cautiously. Each of the roles provides scope for someone to develop as an internal facilitator and to improve the effectiveness of their healthcare organisation and its people.

Key actions

1 It is essential to appreciate that successful OD interventions come in various shapes and sizes, and that one size does not fit all. Find someone in your healthcare organisation to be your adviser who actually understands the various approaches.

2 Managing change effectively is a time-consuming and highly skilled management activity. To be a successful manager (whether you are a general manager or a clinician) you must master the practice of managing change.

3 Develop an OD model, including one for the management of change, that works for you and stick to it. But do not become blinkered – listen to the suggestions of other colleagues. Appoint external consultants with great care, and only when it is clear that such expertise does not exist internally.

4 Practising internal change management is cost-effective and personally rewarding.

REFERENCES

1 Burke WW (1993) *Organization Development: process of learning and changing.* Addison-Wesley, Reading, MA.
2 French WL, Bell CH and Zawacki R (2000) *Organization Development and Transformation.* McGraw-Hill Education, Singapore.
3 Cummings TG and Worley CG (2001) *Organization Development and Change.* Southwestern College Publishing, Cincinnati, OH.
4 Bennis W (1999) *Organization Development.* Addison-Wesley Publishing, Reading, MA.
5 Adams JD (1997) Creating critical mass to support change. In: DF Van Eynde, *et al.* (eds) *Organization Development Classics.* Jossey-Bass, San Francisco, CA.
6 Beckhard R and Harris RT (1987) *Organizational Transitions.* Addison-Wesley, Reading, MA.
7 Hamel G (2000) *Leading the Revolution.* Harvard Business School Press, Boston, MA.
8 Carnall CA (1999) *Managing Change in Organizations.* Pearson Education, Harlow.
9 Senge PM (1990) *The Fifth Discipline: the art and practice of the learning organization.* Century Business, London.
10 Wheatley M (1999) *Leadership and the New Science: discovering order in a chaotic world.* Berrett-Koehler, San Francisco, CA.
11 Kanter RM (1989) *When Giants Learn To Dance.* International Thomson Business Press, London.
12 French WL, Bell CH and Zawacki R (2000) *Organization Development and Transformation.* McGraw-Hill Education, Singapore.
13 Peters T and Waterman R (1982) *In Search of Excellence.* Harper and Row, New York.
14 Senge PM (1990) *The Fifth Discipline: the art and practice of the learning organization.* Century Business, London.
15 Cummings TG and Worley CG (2001) *Organization Development and Change.* Southwestern College Publishing, Cincinnati, OH.
16 Becker BE, Huselid MA and Ulrich D (2001) *The HR Scorecard.* Harvard Business School Press, Boston, MA.
17 Kleiner A, Roberts R, Ross R, *et al.* (1999) The challenge of profound change. In: P Senge, *et al.* (eds.) *The Dance of Change.* Nicholas Brealey, New York.
18 Ulrich D (1996) *Human Resource Champions.* Harvard Business School Press, Boston, MA.
19 Beckhard R and Harris RT (1987) *Organizational Transitions.* Addison-Wesley, Reading, MA.
20 Kotter JP (1996) *Leading Change.* Harvard Business School Press, Boston, MA.
21 These recollections are based on a conference session led by Rosabeth Moss Kanter in Cardiff in 1993.
22 Iles V and Sutherland K (2001) *Organisational Change.* (Managing Change in the NHS). Department of Health, London.
23 Courtney H (2001) *20/20 Foresight: crafting strategy in an uncertain world.* Harvard Business School Press, Boston, MA.
24 Covey SR (1998) Foreword. In: LC Spears (ed.) *Insights on Leadership.* John Wiley and Sons, New York.

CHAPTER 3

The team player

This is the story about four people
Named Everybody, Somebody, Anybody and Nobody.
There was an important job to be done
And Everybody was asked to do it.
Everybody was sure Somebody would do it.
Anybody could have done it
But Nobody did it.
Somebody got angry about that
Because it was Everybody's job.
Everybody thought Anybody could do it
But Nobody realised
That Everybody wouldn't do it.
It ended up
That Everybody blamed Somebody
When Nobody did
What Everybody could have done.[1]

There is a well-known question. Some people say it was asked by Tom Peters, the world-famous management guru, and others claim it was first posed by Peter Senge, the Massachusetts Institute of Technology (MIT) academic and systems expert, but whoever asked it, it's a great question: 'Why is it that team members can have individual IQs of around 150, but when they meet together the team's collective IQ is no more than 68?'

Why is it that a team can agree on a course of action when most, if not all, of the team members claim to disagree with the decision after the meeting has concluded? Many a time I have stood around a coffee pot, or in the car park, after a meeting only to hear members of the team express their disbelief that the meeting could have concluded with such an action plan. Why does this happen?

And why is it that some teams have excellent meetings while others have experiences that leave team members willing to volunteer for anything other than attendance at future meetings? Why do some people adore team meetings while others loathe them? Why are some team members garrulous when asked to contribute at a meeting, while others find the experience of contributing almost excruciatingly painful?

Although there are no simple answers to most of these questions, some of the answers and ways in which to improve team meetings are to be found in straightforward, common-sense approaches to the needs of teams. A number of expert commentators have addressed these principles and their application, and in this chapter I shall draw out key principles and introduce a number of practical observations from my experience as a team member and my work with teams. All of the points I make and the examples I use are taken from my time working in healthcare, and are supported by what I have experienced in other parts of the public sector. These principles and practical observations may cause the response 'But that's obvious!' Is it? Is it obvious? I started this section with a quote by Peters (or was it Senge?) so let me end with one that is definitely by Peters: 'If the obvious is so obvious, then why aren't more people doing it?' If the points I make are that obvious, then I can safely assume that the teams you are running are rich and fulfilling experiences for you and, more importantly, for your colleagues.

WHEN IS A TEAM NOT A TEAM?

My use of the word *team* to cover teams, groups, committees and other collections of people within an organisation may well upset some people, including some pedants who like nothing better than to spend hours defining their terms precisely and debating the differences between a team and other forms of organisational pond-life. I agree that there are often significant variations between teams and groups, and I fully accept that there are times when it is important to understand the differences between the various manifestations of a team (e.g. management team, formal or informal team, top team, self-managing team, project team) and the groups to be found in organisations (e.g. steering committee, advisory board and the group of people you work with under a manager or clinician).

Healthcare managers and clinicians can be helped to reflect on the different types of teams and groups in their organisation, and one device, taken from an academic work,[2] allows the manager or clinician to consider the values, skills and activities of the people involved. Then the people involved can determine whether they are a team or a group! I have to say that, in my experience, most healthcare staff are not too bothered whether they are leading a team or a group. What they require is productive and effective meetings and outcomes that will achieve the purpose behind the establishment of the team or group.

On the occasions when there is a need to arrive at a precise definition of a team, and this may be when the team has a key set of objectives to deliver against a tight time-frame, my favourite definition comes from the seminal work of Katzenbach and Smith:

> A team is a *small number* of people with *complementary skills* who are committed to a *common purpose, performance goals*, and *approach* for which they hold themselves *mutually accountable*.[3]

This elegant definition is extremely useful for leading a team's deliberations. The italicising of six of the terms is not accidental, and Katzenbach and Smith's emphasis on the concepts of size, skills, purpose, goals, approach (or style) and accountability are a line manager's dream, and many a productive hour can be spent assessing the performance of a team against these particular standards. Some of Katzenbach and Smith's concepts may emerge later in this chapter, but at this stage the main issue is the definition of the word *team*.

WHAT'S IN A NAME?

My view on the utility of arriving at a precise definition for each of the terms was made clear earlier on when I referred to pedants and their desire for precision. Experience has taught me that the use of definitions and absolute clarity with regard to the use of the words *teams* or *groups* only has a significant benefit (if any benefit at all) at the start of the session with a team or group. It allows them to think about the different groups of people to which they belong, and to bear in mind that although something may be suitable for one team/group setting it may not be suitable for another team/group setting. Thereafter, I take the view that definitions feed the desires of the pedants and may even exasperate other members of the team, and that there is far more to be gained from working meaningfully with the people, whether they call themselves a team, a group, a committee, a working party, a project board or anything else. The purists (who include among their number many academics) understandably want to differentiate between teams, groups and other gatherings, and may find my view difficult to accommodate. However, the needs of the individuals who belong to these teams, and of their organisations, are so important that what they want is someone who will help them to establish a clear purpose for their activity, help to clarify the roles that they play, help them to understand the dynamics of their meetings and help them to reflect on the effectiveness of their numerous actions. What they need less of is someone who will expound to them the subtle nuances that distinguish a group from a team. The purists are not wrong in their pursuit of precision and definition, but it is the pragmatists who find the greater welcome from healthcare managers and clinicians who have a challenging agenda to deliver.

The point of definition does not end with the difference between a team and a group, but also extends to the habit that many people have of using the terms *teamworking* and *teambuilding* as synonyms. It is important to discuss with colleagues, in a polite and diplomatic way, exactly what they mean by these terms. Many a time I have been asked to help with teambuilding only to discover that the team's greatest need is for someone to help them to identify a 'clarity of purpose' – in other words, to identify the main purpose of their existence. The purists again might debate whether this is the first step in effective teambuilding or effective teamworking, and that is exactly why I prefer not to spend too much time debating and agreeing precise definitions. The important thing, surely, is for senior managers and clinicians to achieve clarity in what they are trying to achieve, and whether that is called *teambuilding* or *teamworking* seems to me to be a secondary consideration.

THE WORK OF TEAMS

Edgar Schein[4] provides a first-class insight into the work of teams (although he refers to them as groups) through what he calls their 'task functions, building and maintenance functions, and boundary management functions'. He lists a range of functions, and in so doing demonstrates the intricacy and breadth of activities associated with team roles. The task functions include information seeking, opinion giving and consensus testing. Building and maintenance functions include standard setting, encouraging and harmonising. Boundary management functions include boundary defining, negotiating and managing entry and exit.

Anyone who is experienced in running a team, or being a member of one, will find most of Schein's terms self-explanatory, and I encourage anyone who wishes to explore this subject further to make themselves conversant with his excellent work. Even for those who are less conversant with these terms, it still remains evident that the range of activities a team has to undertake demonstrates the complexity of its role and the difficulty in performing them effectively.

The complex and critically important role of teams is also demonstrated in the work of Ken Blanchard,[5] who consistently manages to bring together research, management experience and common sense and a down-to-earth approach. Through the use of the acronym 'PERFORM' he identifies the characteristics of high-performing teams as: **P**urpose, **E**mpowerment, **R**elationships and communication, **F**lexibility, **O**ptimal productivity, **R**ecognition and appreciation and **M**orale. On the basis of his PERFORM acronym Blanchard has constructed a useful team diagnostic instrument to test the extent to which teams are meeting these criteria.

These glimpses from the work of Schein and Blanchard (and there are many other analysts with important contributions to make in this area) demonstrate a fundamentally important point about teams. The role that teams are asked to undertake in a healthcare organisation is often complex, often extensive and broad in its range of activities, and unless these teams are handled expertly they are likely to be an unsatisfactory experience for their members and an ineffective activity for the organisations that have established them. Schein and Blanchard demonstrate this to be the case, as do the writings of Katzenbach and Smith and many other authors.

THE IMPORTANCE OF TEAMS

This gives rise to a fundamental question. If teams are such important dimensions of organisational life, why is it that so many of them give the appearance of having been thrown together without too much thought, are serviced in a way that does not help them to deliver their objectives, possess a lack of clarity as to what is expected of them, and contain members who would rather be doing something else? Conversely, why are some healthcare teams wonderful experiences that energise their members, deliver results ahead of time, and are fulfilling experiences in every sense of the phrase?

Let me start with the negative experiences. I remember well belonging to a health authority management team chaired by a chief executive (in those days they were called district general managers). It met at 2.00 pm on the first Tuesday of each month, and although its terms of reference claimed that its role was to provide strategic leadership to the health authority and its hospital general managers, its agenda was dominated by operational activities, often trifling ones that meant it never concluded its deliberations until some time between 8.30 and 9.00 pm. To make matters worse, every month the chief executive would aggressively challenge and seemingly attempt to humiliate one of the members of the team. This confrontation usually took place some time between 6.00 and 6.30 pm, and the team members were convinced that it was induced by a substantial lack of caffeine and nicotine and the interaction of this with what some saw as a somewhat malevolent personality. I was lucky in that the outburst was only directed at me on one occasion, but some colleagues appeared to be regular recipients. The meetings were dreaded by most of the team (*sic*) members.

Another team to which I belonged, in another healthcare organisation, had been established to oversee the implementation of a major information technology (IT) infrastructure. I had been invited to join the team to contribute an organisation development perspective to its deliberations. It recognised, or so it claimed, that its strategy should not be IT-driven ('IT is only the vehicle to achieve our business objectives', it claimed), but that IT should be a response to the overarching needs of the organisation (I can still remember the jargon!). The reality was that the team meetings became a paradise for the nerds and anoraks of IT, and the discussions, which included numerous acronyms and technical terms, fuelled the intensity with which they bandied about their latest thinking. The fact that I felt like a visitor to a foreign country is only important in the context that the meeting was supposed to be about the overall strategy of the organisation, but had in fact become little more than a technical-reporting session.

Another negative experience will hopefully reinforce the point. I was invited to observe the meetings of the executive management team of an NHS trust well known in its part of the country. The chief executive, a splendid person and very good company, was concerned that the team was not as effective as he had hoped. He thought that an outside pair of eyes might be able to spot the problem and advise him how to make things more effective. I arrived at the meetings and could hardly believe my eyes. The meeting did not start on time, some people turned up late, the agenda contained 18 items, many of which were low-level operational matters, and some of the papers were tabled and had not been considered by the members. I saw two members removing the agenda and papers from the envelope for what appeared to be the first time, members failed to understand the importance and/or urgency of the agenda and allowed relatively unimportant items to drag on indefinitely and, worst of all, it became clear that the chief executive, director of finance and one other person had already been through the agenda and agreed the outcome of every important agenda item. The result of this was an ineffective team meeting. Many of the so-called team members realised that the agenda had been 'carved up' before the start of the meeting, and they were convinced that they were in fact wasting their time.

These are just three anecdotes to make the point that many team meetings are negative experiences. Thankfully, most are first-class experiences.

GREAT TEAM MEETINGS

I remember joining one NHS team that turned out to be one of the most rewarding work experiences of my life. There were eight of us in the team, and in many ways it was the perfect match. We represented a mixture of ages and gender, our work experiences were varied, our personalities seemed to gel rather than clash, and the 'big-picture' individuals were more than compensated for by those who were determined to produce and deliver a project plan. The team was perfect, and we worked together closely for many years and remain good friends to this day. We worked hard, but we also managed to have fun. Looking back on those days, the success of the team was partly down to the way in which it had been put together and to the way in which it was led, and partly down to some good luck, but above all it was due to the members who were personally committed to the project in hand and totally driven to make sure that it was seen as an overwhelming triumph.

Another memorable experience involved me sitting as a director of another health authority. The various healthcare activities represented around the boardroom table were diverse, but there was a unity of spirit, partly caused by adversity (times were tough) and partly due to the quality of the chief executive who brought the various activities together under a coherent framework and ran the authority in a way that allowed established functions to thrive as well as providing an incubator in which new activities could grow. We worked hard but we also had a good time together and, over time, we were seen as a successful enterprise. The authority had a clear mission statement and set of values, it provided a range of quality services that represented value for money, and its people were seen to be professional.

FIVE COMMON FEATURES OF SUCCESSFUL HEALTHCARE TEAMS

As I think back to those and many other experiences of successful team membership in healthcare, five common features emerge to explain why they were positive and effective experiences.

1 They have a clear sense of purpose and direction

This sense of purpose and direction was shared by all of the team's members. That may seem to be an obvious and basic point, but I have been in teams where there was a lack of clarity about what it was the team was being asked to deliver. Similarly, I have been a part of a team where the purpose was clear but certain members, often without overtly revealing their position, were opposed to the purpose of the team or usually because of their affiliation to some other team or professional body (including trade unions), or for personal reasons. It is essential that the team understands what they are required to do, that they know the parameters in which they have to function, that they know when they have to deliver the results required and that they are all, without reservation or condition, signed up to the purpose of the team.

2 They have openness as a key characteristic

Members of these teams felt that they were able to say what they thought (a situation that certainly does not exist in some so-called teams, where an unguarded comment can have dire consequences) and that their different views of the world were positively encouraged by the leader. This openness meant that opposing viewpoints were seen as being quite legitimate and a means of moving towards the 'truth' about a particular situation. This led to a decrease in conflict, to the point where it is hard to remember anything other than harmonious relationships and an increase in imaginative and rounded decisions. Life in a team where there is no fear of retribution is a truly liberating experience. There are times, of course, when a team member can take advantage of such liberty and abuse the freedom by turning it into a licence for unacceptable behaviour. It is difficult when a colleague is being unjustifiably negative or critical over a prolonged period, especially when this is being driven by personal reasons originating outside the workplace. Such situations have to be dealt with by the chair of the team. However, an open environment that may allow some problems to intrude is far better than a closed environment in which creative thought is stifled due to fear of reprisal.

Another aspect of openness in team affairs is the opportunity for learning through reflection. Reflection is critical from time to time, and many of my former colleagues would contend that reflection should be a part of each and every team agenda. There is a simple question for all teams to address: 'How are we doing?' In my files I have retained a quote from a colleague and fellow team member on this need for learning (although he or she must forgive me for no longer remembering who it was that actually said it):

> I believe you have to make learning a conscious thing, if you want to make the team effective. You have to address it as an issue, putting time aside to work on learning issues and recognise that it is as important as achieving objectives. It is critical that a team comes to understand and view itself as a learning body.

Openness demands such an approach and, through discussion at the end of the meeting or with the aid of some diagnostic technique and/or the help of an internal change agent or facilitator, making time available for learning and reflection can have a considerable payback.

3 They have a balanced membership

By this I mean they were teams made up of people who saw the world differently, who had complementary skills and backgrounds, with a variety of personalities and ages, and who gave the team energy and enthusiasm. All too often team members appear to be clones of one another (*The Attack of the Clones* is not just a Star Wars film); and having a team that has balance, or at the very least a team that is aware of where it might be out of kilter, is essential. Far too often teams are made up of 'like-minded people', colleagues who 'won't rock the boat', and those who have served in teams, most probably called committees, for so long that they have developed a language that sounds like an acrid set of minutes, and so miss the dynamism that a well-constructed team can generate. Gary Hamel,[6] with his usual wit, expressed a similar view on the formulation of strategy in many organisations:

> in most companies strategy is the preserve of the old guard. Strategy conversations have the same 10 people talking to the same 10 people year after year. No wonder the strategies that emerge are dull as dishwater . . . they've been talking at each other for years – their positions are well rehearsed, they can finish each other's sentences.

I have sat in on meetings where a team is being put together, and although it was always the case that members were considered on the basis of their professional background, geographical location, gender and race, departmental function, (occasionally) track record and availability, I can barely remember an instance where the composition of the team was an issue of complementarity based on factors such as their preferred role within a team and individual personality.

Creating teams

Establishing a balanced team is not that difficult, and there are many ways in which a manager can be helped to do this. Meredith Belbin's work is famous. Over a period of nine years, he and his associates observed the behaviour of large numbers of managers from across the world as they participated in a Henley Management College programme. As the Belbin website[7] explains, 'their different core personality traits, intellectual styles and behaviours were assessed [and] as time progressed different clusters of behaviour were identified as underlying the success of the teams. These successful clusters were then given names.' The nine traditional behaviours are shown in Figure 3.1, and the differences in personality and in their contribution to a team between, for example, the plant (creative, imaginative, unorthodox) and the completer finisher (painstaking, conscientious, anxious, searches out errors) are familiar to anyone who has been a member of a team. If this is known, then why are so many teams full of *plants*, who find it hard to get anything done but who have a wonderful time exploring new ideas, or *completer finishers*, who can produce first-class project plans but who have few ideas to project manage. There are many examples of imbalanced teams that could be cited, but the one that stands out above all the others comes from a former colleague of mine who spent a nearly suicidal afternoon trying to encourage a team of internal auditors to act creatively. Enough said.

The Myers-Briggs Type Indicator (MBTI), which is discussed in greater detail in Chapter 9 on personal growth, is another valuable tool when discussing the importance of self-awareness and its significance to team membership. Understanding how individuals with a preference for *extraversion* or *introversion* are energised; how those who prefer *sensing* to *intuition* take in information; how *thinkers* and *feelers* arrive at a decision, and how those with a preference for *perceiving* as opposed to *judging* relate to the world around them has a major part to play in determining the effectiveness of a team. It is unethical, according to

Belbin team-role type	Contributions	Allowable weaknesses
PLANT PL	Creative, imaginative, unorthodox. Solves difficult problems	Ignores incidentals. Too preoccupied to communicate effectively
CO-ORDINATOR CO	Mature, confident, a good chairperson. Clarifies goals, promotes decision-making, delegates well	Can often be seen as manipulative. Offloads personal work
MONITOR EVALUATOR ME	Sober, strategic and discerning. Sees all options. Judges accurately	Lacks drive and ability to inspire others
IMPLEMENTER IMP	Disciplined, reliable, conservative and efficient. Turns ideas into practical actions	Somewhat inflexible. Slow to respond to new ideas
COMPLETER FINISHER CF	Painstaking, conscientious, anxious. Searches out errors and omissions. Delivers on time	Inclined to worry unduly. Reluctant to delegate
RESOURCE INVESTIGATOR RI	Extrovert, enthusiastic, communicative. Explores opportunities. Develops contacts	Over-optimistic. Loses interest once initial enthusiasm has passed
SHAPER SH	Challenging, dynamic, thrives on pressure. The drive and courage to overcome obstacles	Prone to provocation. Offends people's feelings
TEAMWORKER TW	Co-operative, mild, perceptive and diplomatic. Listens, builds, averts friction	Indecisive in crunch situations
SPECIALIST SP	Single-minded, self-starting, dedicated. Provides knowledge and skills in rare supply	Contributes only on a narrow front. Dwells on technicalities

FIGURE 3.1 Belbin's team roles

the guardians of the MBTI, to use the tool as a device for recruitment and selection, but in terms of understanding a team and working towards complementary roles it has a great deal to offer. If there is an awareness that a colleague may sometimes, or even often, act only in accordance with their personality type in a team meeting, or even counter to their personality type when experiencing significant levels of stress, there is an opportunity for meaningful teambuilding activities. One healthcare organisation in which a colleague of mine worked even went to the length of inviting its senior employees (the invitation was a genuine one and respected fully the need for confidentiality) to wear their four MBTI letters on a badge – 'I'm an ENTP' or 'I'm an ISTJ', or any of the other 14 variations. This provided many opportunities for good-natured leg-pulling and, most importantly, opportunities for development in the effectiveness of the various teams. Although a preference should not be viewed as a debilitating factor, it does provide useful insights into how someone may well respond.

4 *They focus their attention on performance*

Teams may have a far from perfect balance in terms of membership, or they may be experiencing difficulties in finding time for reflection and learning, but having a focus on performance is a non-negotiable variable, a *sine qua non* or indispensable condition when it comes to effectiveness. Without it, the team will paddle around in a sea of options without recognising the urgency and importance of their task. With it, they are more likely to be focused and deliver against the deadlines and targets that have been set for the task.

The work of Katzenbach and Smith[8] illustrates the importance of the focus on performance: 'Significant performance challenges energise teams regardless of where they are in an organisation' and 'organisational leaders can foster team performance best by building a strong performance ethic rather than by establishing a team-promoting environment alone'. These are significant points that are of consequence to managers who are wrestling with difficult team members or with teams which are finding it difficult to achieve a sense of urgency in their work. One of my colleagues headed a healthcare team that included a member who was expert at obfuscating most discussions, raising irrelevant issues and showing his disdain for many of the alternative courses of action under consideration. The team member had been foisted upon this manager, and his removal was not an available option. Furthermore, his unhelpful behaviour was exhibited in such a way that he could justify it as being a genuine enquiry and the consideration of potential alternative options. We knew him to be a member of the 'awkward squad', and would willingly have ejected him from the team. The answer to this problem member was to focus on performance – everything became performance driven, all attempts by him to deviate were thwarted and, over time and despite his actions, the team achieved its objectives.

Top teams

The performance of teams at the top of an organisation deserves special attention. When I work with senior executive teams to help to make their team more effective, it is easy to see that they would not welcome suggestions that they should engage in activities which they would consider 'warm and cosy' with the explicit (or even implicit) intention of making them into a team whose members actually enjoyed one another's company. There is usually laughter when I assure them that team effectiveness does not mean that they will have to like each other, or climb a mountain together, or go off and have a curry each Friday evening before leaving for home. Behind the laughter the relief is palpable. These are senior people who have climbed the greasy pole to the top of the organisational tree. They have got there by being single-minded, highly motivated, self-disciplined, and perhaps even a little selfish. The last thing they want is some outsider attempting to turn them into a fluffy, cuddly, team-loving individual. They want to achieve – they crave better performance so that their own position may be enhanced.

Again Katzenbach's work is relevant. He shows that at the highest level in an organisation the use of the phrase *top team* may not refer to a team in the usual sense of the term at all:

> The CEO invariably functions as the single leader of a group whose membership is based on formal positions rather than on individual skills, whose purpose and goals are indistinguishable from the overall corporate purpose and goals, and whose behaviours are determined entirely by individual accountability.

His book, *Teams at the Top*,[9] has important messages to illustrate the peculiar place of top teams, the best ways in which they can maximise performance, and how they should operate, both within and outside team settings, in accordance with the needs of the organisation.

5 They have an effective leader who adopts an appropriate leadership style

Life would be so much easier for all of us if it were possible to list the attributes that an effective team leader should possess and then to coach individuals to become competent at each of them. We all know that organisational life in healthcare is sometimes not that easy, yet some management texts are written in a style which suggests that most management tasks are straightforward – the books give the impression that all teams and team members are identical, and that mastery of the competencies contained in the books will ensure the transformation of the team that is being led. However, life is not that simple. Teams differ, team members differ (individual team members can even react differently within and between meetings), the issues being dealt with call for different approaches, the culture of the organisation may dictate certain approaches, there are times when a participative style or a more directional leadership style is appropriate, and time pressures may mean that there are occasions when a less than subtle position has to be taken. This means that simplistic lists can be used for guidance but they must never be seen as a template for action in all types of circumstances. There are pointers – general principles – that can be used to increase the effectiveness of team leaders, but they are only of value when used selectively and by someone who understands the issues surrounding the dynamics of a team. Even with that substantial caveat I shall resist the temptation to provide a list of suggestions for effective team leadership. To do so would duplicate the work of many other writers who have provided such advice, and would also appear to be a contradiction of the main point I have made, namely that effective team leadership must be sensitive to the circumstances under which the team is led, and the diagnosis and application of a successful style of leadership takes far more than the application of six or seven competences that have been picked up in a management textbook. I intend no criticism of the distinguished writers on the leadership of teams, and I encourage the reader to consult their books and manuals. However, the major point, and a point on which I believe those writers would concur, is that developing and applying the most appropriate style of team leadership, or team membership and teamworking, requires expert help and is not something that should be treated superficially.

Key actions

1 Do not get 'hung up' about whether you belong to a team, group or committee, but instead concentrate on the contribution that is expected from you and what you have to do to be seen to be an effective member.
2 Teams have important contributions to make, and membership of a team is usually a rewarding experience. If your team is going through difficult times, the best way through that difficulty is to concentrate on matters of performance.
3 Although there are common features shared by successful teams, do not fall into the trap of believing that one approach will work with all teams. Leading a team calls for vigilance, attention to detail and the nurturing of individual team members.

REFERENCES

1 Doppler K and Lauterburg CH (2001) *Managing Corporate Change*. Springer-Verlag, Berlin.
2 Leigh A and Maynard M (2002) *Leading Your Team*. Nicholas Brealey, London.
3 Katzenbach JR and Smith DK (1998) *The Wisdom of Teams*. McGraw Hill, Maidenhead.
4 Schein EH (1988) *Process Consultation: its role in organizational development. Volume 1*. Addison Wesley, Reading, MA.
5 Blanchard K, Carew D and Parisi-Carew E (1996) *One-Minute Manager Builds High Performing Teams*. HarperCollins Business, London.
6 Hamel G (2000) *Leading the Revolution*. Harvard Business School Press, Boston, MA.
7 www.belbin.com
8 Katzenbach JR and Smith DK (1998) *Wisdom of Teams*. McGraw-Hill, Maidenhead.
9 Katzenbach JR (1998) *Teams at the Top*. Harvard Business School Press, Boston, MA.

CHAPTER 4

Organisational learning: can the right hand know what the left hand is doing?

My wife Lesley works as a speech and language adviser for our local education authority and with children with special needs in a local school. The children she works with are sometimes very intelligent, sometimes less intelligent than average (whatever the term 'average' is taken to mean), and most of the children are just typical kids. The one thing that brings them together, and categorises them as special-needs children, is that they have a particular (speech and language) learning difficulty. These days the experts know enough about Asperger's Syndrome, dyslexia and other conditions to realise that it is a learning difficulty that can be addressed and that it is not some overwhelming debilitating condition. There are sufficient examples of outstandingly successful people with Asperger's or dyslexia to prove that having this not an insurmountable obstacle. How different from times gone by. When I was at school, most children with dyslexia (a condition that was generally undiagnosed and unappreciated at that time, of course) were patronised and considered to be 'slow' or even referred to as 'thick' by the teachers, and were then given a clip around the ear to encourage them to deal with their 'thickness' or 'stupidity'. Thank goodness times have changed and that special-needs experts, even if they may only understand a fraction of what will become self-evident in a century's time, are able to cater for the learning requirements of this particular group of children.

'What does all of this have to do with healthcare organisational life?' you might be thinking. I contend that there are clear similarities, and that in the world of work – and that includes the healthcare sector and the remainder of the public services – a transformation is taking place. The use of knowledge, the benefits of learning and the concept of intellectual capital are becoming of paramount importance, yet there are some organisations, and key individuals within those organisations, who have special learning needs. They need to think differently, to understand how they and their organisations should learn, and it is essential that someone addresses their learning disabilities as a matter of urgency, otherwise they are not going to make the progress that they ought to make. The radical transformation taking place means that the importance of knowledge and learning and the ability to challenge the status quo with new and different ways of thinking has become a critical factor in the future success of all healthcare organisations. When I speak to healthcare managers and clinicians about these issues, they voice agreement with the urgency of action required in these areas.

THE EVIDENCE

Think about these words from Pope John Paul II in his 1991 encyclical *Centesimus Annus*:

> Whereas at one time the decisive factor of production was the land, and later capital . . . today the decisive factor is increasingly man himself, that is, his knowledge.[1]

Or consider these words, from a less exalted person admittedly, who in a description of the Third Wave (the title he attaches to the knowledge revolution) shows the rapidity of change that is being experienced:

> Humanity faces a quantum leap forward. It faces the deepest social upheaval and creative restructuring of all time. Without clearly recognising it, we are engaged in building a remarkable new civilisation from the ground up. This is the meaning of the Third Wave. Until now the human race has undergone two great waves of change . . . The first wave of change – the agricultural revolution – took thousands of years to play itself out. The second wave – the rise of industrial civilisation – took a mere three hundred years. Today history is even more accelerative, and it is likely that the Third Wave will sweep across history and complete itself in a few decades.[2]

Or consider these words from the intellectual capital guru Thomas A Stewart, who shows the change at the very heart of the employment relationship:

> The rise of the knowledge worker fundamentally alters the nature of work and the agenda of management. Managers are custodians; they protect and care for the assets of a corporation; when the assets are intellectual, the manager's job changes. Knowledge work doesn't happen the way mechanical labour did.[3]

Think of your own experiences in healthcare and beyond. If someone had said to me, as little as 10 years ago, that I would spend much of my time working behind a laptop, with remote access to an NHS and then a university computer system, and the opportunity to travel almost anywhere via my Toshiba, I would not have believed them. Yet the transformation is taking place and we need little persuasion, no matter how carefully chosen the quotes, to prove that we live in days of breathtaking change. It truly is both fascinating and scary – and the successful people in terms of work, but not necessarily in terms of all other aspects of life, are those who make sure that they are not being left behind. The sensible healthcare organisations are those that make sure they understand the importance of developing the concept of intellectual capital; of incorporating the concept of knowledge management; of seeing learning, thinking and reflection as key organisational competencies; and of being open to the ideas of those who once might have been seen as corporate rebels. Understanding these ideas in greater detail and meeting the challenges that arise from them are essential.

THE POWER OF ORGANISATIONAL LEARNING

Peter Senge is one of the doyens of organisational learning. His landmark book *The Fifth Discipline*[4] was seen as one of the most influential books on organisations and their people of the twentieth century, and his influential Society for Organisational Learning (SOL) has offshoots in countries around the world. I have to declare one minor interest in that I am a member of SOL UK. It meets four or five times a year, has the opportunity to listen to senior figures from a variety of backgrounds describe their attempts to take forward learning in their organisations, and the commitment to Senge's teachings might be seen by some to resemble the practice of cult members!

Definitions abound on the meaning of organisational learning, or the learning organisation, and although it is important to be able to describe what is meant by these terms, I take the view that an exact definition is less important than a commitment to the ideals it embodies. To quote the old Scottish preacher 'It is better felt than telt'.

Nevertheless, here are two helpful definitions of the organisational learning concept. Senge's definition of such a state is one of them:

> Where people continually expand their capacity to create the results they truly desire, where new expansive patterns of thinking are nurtured, where collective aspiration is set free, and where people are continually learning how to learn together.[5]

Most other definitions state similar concepts in similar words, although some emphasise individual aspects of the wider definition. The other helpful definition comes from David Garvin:

> A learning organisation is an organisation skilled at creating, acquiring, interpreting, transferring and retaining knowledge, and at purposefully modifying its behaviour to reflect new knowledge and insights.[6]

Once the important hurdle of understanding the definition has been overcome, the next step is to understand the components needed to work towards being able to describe one's healthcare organisation as a learning organisation. I use the phrase *work towards* as it would be a very brave or foolish individual who would claim to have fully arrived at a complete state of learning. I am impressed by many writers in this area, and in my experience those that offer practitioners the greatest support are the writings of Richard Beckhard and Wendy Pritchard[7] and, inevitably, Peter Senge.[8]

Beckhard and Pritchard show that a learning organisation that is functioning well has several elements in place, including a clear picture of how the organisation should operate, feedback systems that guarantee ongoing information, information systems designed to support the balance between performing and doing, training and education programmes, a communication strategy and a strategic planning process and strategic objectives that include learning.

Peter Senge, in applying his organisational learning definition, puts forward the view that:

> Today, I believe, five new 'component technologies' are gradually converging to innovate learning organisations. Though developed separately, each will, I believe, prove critical to the others' success, just as occurs with any ensemble. Each provides a vital dimension in building organisations that can truly 'learn', that can continually enhance their capacity to realise their highest aspirations.

From this position he goes on to set out his exceptionally well-known five dimensions, and he explains their composition and interrelationship. The five dimensions (abbreviated to the briefest possible format) are as follows:

➤ *systems thinking* – to recognise 'invisible fabrics of interrelated actions'
➤ *personal mastery* – 'deepening our personal vision'
➤ *mental models* – 'those deeply ingrained assumptions'
➤ *building shared vision* – 'the capacity to hold a shared picture of the future'
➤ *team learning* – 'ways to stimulate learning'.

Senge builds upon these dimensions, and his perceptive *11 Laws of the Fifth Discipline* (e.g. today's problems arise from yesterday's 'solutions') and his *7 Learning Disabilities* (e.g. the parable of the boiled frog, which is a must for all readers) make fascinating reading and ought to challenge every leader to examine practices in their healthcare organisation. I also believe that Senge's writing on how leaders can build a learning organisation[9] should become essential reading (and not just for those with an interest in the subject), and his description of the importance of 'aspiration', 'reflective conversation' and 'complexity' is of special importance to all those involved in healthcare organisations.

Organisational learning: two healthcare examples

Beckhard, Pritchard and Senge have set out what many will see as a convincing argument, but the question still remains about what happens in practice. I do not want to suggest that there is an overwhelming resistance to learning in all organisational environments – there are many examples of the adoption of best practice – but the following two real-life examples of a learning disability are all too common. The examples are taken from two healthcare organisations, but some of the facts have been changed to protect the identity of those organisations. They are true stories, and two examples of the unsuccessful adoption of organisational learning have been chosen, as they are more informative.

Organisation A asked me to work with them on what they called *top team development*. This was an assignment to work with the top 30 or so senior managers in the organisation and to address the development needs of the senior staff. I spent a considerable amount of time working with them on an individual basis and got to know most of them fairly well. We reached a position where we could trust one another and they knew that anything they said to me on a confidential basis would remain a confidence. After this comprehensive series of one-to-one discussions, we arranged to meet together for a single day at a local hotel. In fact the sessions were seen to be so productive by the participants that we met on three occasions over a six-month period. As I fed back what I had discovered through the one-to-one interviews (there was an unsurprising consistency in the views that everyone had expressed to me) and we debated the issues in a plenary session, one key action emerged. The delegates all agreed that one of their monthly management meetings had become far too operational in nature, the agenda had become ridiculously long, and they all felt that the majority of the time spent in this meeting should be devoted to learning from experience (reflection) and to some aspect of personal or team development. As an action point it was agreed that in future the morning of the meeting would be devoted to learning and development, and the afternoon to important or urgent operational issues. A new world order was dawning for this executive team. This new way of running the meetings was agreed unanimously. They invited me to become an observer at their first meeting, and at the end of their meeting they invited me to feed back some observations. The day of the meeting arrived, and when we met it was clear that the agenda was in two parts. The first part went very well, even though there was a certain understandable awkwardness in handling learning and development issues. The chair of the meeting, the most senior of the executives, was very nervous throughout (in fact I had never seen him so edgy), but he concluded that the whole process had been a most valuable experience, both for individuals and for the organisation. The afternoon was spent looking at three or four major operational matters, and when I gave my feedback it was well received and I was later complimented by many of those present. I took my leave of them feeling rather pleased with myself.

About three months later I made contact with some of the senior staff to ask how the new meetings were going. 'Very well' was the reply, and they explained that they had made one alteration to the arrangements – the morning and after-noon sessions had been swapped. Now they did the operational items in the morning and the learning and development in the afternoon. Things were going very well, they assured me, but there were times when the morning's agenda spilled over into the afternoon, though they were still finding sufficient time to engage in learning and development work together.

After another three months or so I made contact with them again. Yes, you've guessed it, they told me that there had been some other changes. The opera-tional agenda had grown so rapidly and become so pressing that they now had to address this for most of the day, and by the time they got to the late afternoon there wasn't too much enthusiasm for a learning, reflection and development session.

The reality was that a morning devoted to learning and development which they had all seen as an essential was now off the agenda. It was not that it had become unimportant, or that they were unable to carry it out (they had a very able team of in-house development people). It was just that they had found the whole thing to be an uncomfortable experience and had returned to what they did best – dealing with operational issues. Many of them had the good grace to acknowledge this fact and to look up to the heavens with a smile that seemed to say 'But what did you expect' when I met them next.

Organisation B decided that it should become a learning organisation. One of the organisation's directors had attended a management conference and had become convinced that the principles of a learning organisation were exactly what they required for the next stage of their organisation's development. In turn, the other directors and the chief executive eventually became convinced, and as I was already working with them on another long-standing organisation development issue, they asked me if I would provide some support. One of the first things they wished to do was to invite the expert on learning organisations who had spoken at the conference, a very well-known and highly regarded individual, to visit them and discuss the implications of becoming such an organisation. They arranged the meeting, and when it eventually took place (after some initial and alarming pitfalls that, in and of themselves, are a lesson in dealing with false and unrealistic expectations on the part of the organisation), the organisation finally reached a position where it could confidently announce to its large workforce that it had become a learning organisation. The new-found status was also announced in its various corporate strategies and its annual report.

I continued to work with them, although only tangentially on organisation learning, and I could tell from the expressions on the faces of many of the senior staff that either they were not absolutely sure what their newly acquired status actually meant or, if they did understand it, they were not too sure about its relevance to the needs of the organisation.

About 18 months after their announcement that they had *become a learning organisation*, they decided to merge some of the departments in their organisation, both to achieve benefits for patients and to reduce their administrative overheads. Two years previously, and before they had become a *learning organisation*, they had also merged some other departments in another part of their organisation. As they worked on developing and promulgating the merger plans, I was asked to help with some of the organisation development/change management issues. One of the first things I asked, rather naively I now realise, was whether they had taken into account what they could learn from their previous experience of merging operational units. After all, that merger experience was only about three years old, and surely those experiences could help them to successfully implement this merger. The look on their faces said it all. They saw that as something quite unrelated, and dismissed my suggestion with a 'that was handled by another part of the organisation'-type comment. The expression on my face must have revealed how astonished I was. Here was a *learning organisation* that was unable and, more importantly, unwilling to learn from another part of its own organisation. It was not appropriate to press my point with this particular audience, but I did manage to convince some of the senior staff that, at the very least, a learning organisation should be able to learn from its own past experiences. Although the senior managers were convinced of the theory of what I had to say, it became clear that the practice of merging was not always informed by previous learning. It was a startling example of the old adage that what you do and what you say are not always the same thing.

I do not wish to suggest that these two examples are in any way typical of all or even most healthcare organisations, but I do contend that they are typical of far too many organisations, and that there is a need for them to be helped to overcome their learning disability.

Some learning choices

The diagram by Grint[10] shown in Figure 4.1 illustrates the alternatives that are being offered to organisations. In the diagram the choice is between being a 'Sweep-It-Under-The-Carpet-Manager' or one that values the benefits that flow from truly being a learning organisation.

Mayo and Lank's[11] work shows that it is possible to develop what they call a *complete learning organisation*, where a supportive culture and learning climate are generated through the integration of policy and strategy, leadership, people management processes and information technology. This in turn promotes personal learning, team learning and networks and the organisational learning which, so they claim, create value in the organisation. It is fascinating work and certainly worth reading.

Against Mayo and Lank's confident assertion there is empirical and anecdotal evidence to show that some healthcare organisations need to learn how to learn. They need to understand that there are issues associated with the success of the organisation that are directly related to their willingness to be open to new ideas, how they learn from their successes and failures, and how they allow their staff the freedom to experiment with new and improved ways of doing things.

Arie de Geus

Arie de Geus retired from the Royal Dutch/Shell Group in 1989. At that time he held the post of group planning co-ordinator, and had become well known for developing the application of scenario planning within Shell. Since his retirement his work on organisational learning has benefited many. His best-known book, *The Living Company*,[12] highlights the mortality rate of a high proportion of firms by showing that, at the time of his writing, one-third of the 1970 list of *Fortune 500* companies had been acquired or broken into pieces, or had merged with other companies. This high mortality rate led him to pose the question 'Why do so many companies die young?' His answer is fascinating:

> Mounting evidence suggests that corporations fail because their policies and practices are based too heavily on the thinking and the language of economics. Put another way, companies die because their managers focus exclusively on producing goods and services and forget that the organisation is a community of human beings that is in business – any business – to stay alive. Managers concern themselves with land, labour and capital, and overlook the fact that labour means real people.
>
> . . . What I have come to call *living companies* have a personality that allows them to evolve harmoniously. They know who they are, understand how they fit into the world, value new ideas and new people, and husband their money

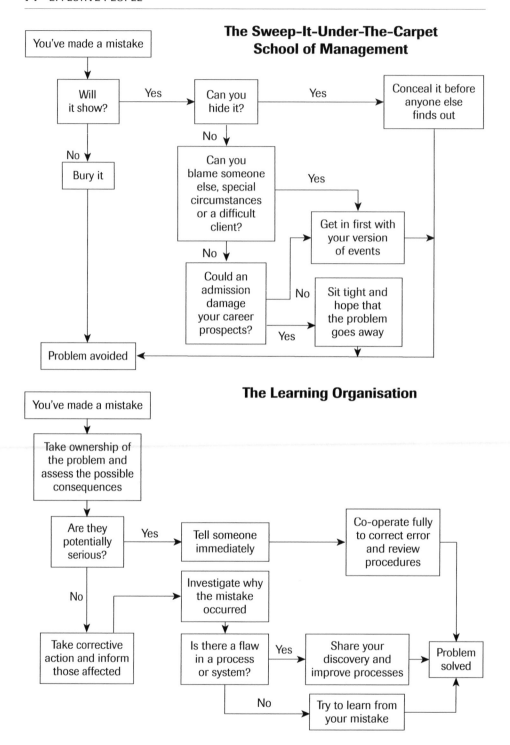

FIGURE 4.1 The non-learning and learning organisation: operational cycle
Source: Grint K (1996) The non-learning and learning organisation. In:
B Garratt (ed.) *The Fish Rots from the Head*. HarperCollins Business, London.

in a way that allows them to govern their future. Those personality traits manifest themselves in behaviours designed to renew the company over many generations.

He demonstrates comprehensively and conclusively the benefits of being a learning organisation, and the lessons are plain for all to see. The conclusion is quite simple – learning is essential and profitable to the development of the organisation. It can also be fun.

KNOWLEDGE MANAGEMENT AND INTELLECTUAL CAPITAL

Two of the history topics I studied as a schoolboy were the agricultural and industrial revolutions. I can still remember learning about the transformation that took place as a result of the exploits of men like 'Turnip' Townsend and Thomas Coke, who 'began to grow wheat, barley, turnips and clover in succession without the need for a fallow year'.[13] Coke also used 'clay and chalk to make the ground more fertile' and used selective breeding to improve the yield and quality of meat and wool. Then there was the wonderfully named Jethro Tull (a name later used by a 1960s rock band), who invented a seed drill that allowed seed to be planted more economically and the ground to be hoed properly. The Industrial Revolution also had its set of heroes, and produced people whose fame has lasted to the present day. Who can forget the name of James Watt and his improved steam engine, or James Hargreaves and the 'spinning jenny', or Samuel Crompton and his 'mule', or Sir Richard Arkwright and his skill in bringing about change in administrative systems?

Our history teacher brought these characters to life and made the respective revolutions as vivid as the French or American Revolutions even to the point that, as schoolboys, we thought that Hargreaves and his associates had one day woken up and thought 'Let's start a revolution!' As my understanding of the agricultural and industrial revolutions developed, I realised that they could not be restricted to a particular time and place in history, and that their effect continued, and in some ways continues still, over centuries. I also came to understand that the effect of these two revolutions was dramatic and had both a positive and also often a negative impact* on the lives of all those concerned with the changes that were taking place. Anyone who is aware of the changes taking place in the economy of China in recent times will understand that the movement from their agricultural and centrally planned system is, in effect, an industrial revolution of the twenty-first century.

---

* I need to acknowledge that there were many downsides to the advances brought by the Industrial Revolution. As a former industrial relations and labour history student, I am only too aware of the problems and of the appalling conditions in many of the factories, but I also contend that to have ignored the developments heralded by the Industrial Revolution would have caused far more problems for the economic prosperity of this country and its people. It would have left any country with a 'peasantry' – a word that has no pejorative connotations in my mind – and future developments in education, health and the overall standard of living would not have taken place.

In much the same way as the agricultural and industrial revolutions brought about substantial change in earlier centuries, developed economies these days are experiencing a third revolution, namely the knowledge revolution. No one can place an exact starting date on it – a Gates or even a Babbage-type character did not sit up one day and say 'I'm going to start a knowledge revolution!' – but it is an incontrovertible fact that developed economies are living through a phenomenal degree of change, and that the change is being driven by the knowledge revolution. Knowledge has become power in much the same way that land, labour and financial capital once were. Although this is far more evident in some communities than in others, the evidence from informed commentators shows that the revolution heralded by the information age, with its equivalents of the Townsends, Tulls and Arkwrights, is impacting across the world. This revolution has many spectacular benefits, but its greatest difficulty lies in people understanding exactly what it will mean for them, how it will change their lives and what impact it will have on their children's careers and lives, and in dealing with a host of other uncertainties. Some people even have one eye on films such as *The Matrix*, a film in which the machines take over the world, and many are understandably apprehensive and concerned about what it will all mean for them. No doubt our ancestors, and the people of China and similar countries today, had or have the same worries. But life goes on inexorably, it seems.

Knowledge revolution definitions

What exactly do the experts mean when they talk about knowledge being the source of a new revolution? Knowledge gurus Thomas Davenport and Laurence Prusak provide what they rather humbly call a working definition rather than a definitive definition of knowledge. They emphasise that their definition expresses the characteristics that make knowledge valuable as well as the characteristics (often the same ones) that make it difficult to manage well:

> Knowledge is a fluid mix of framed experience, values, contextual information and expert insight that provides a framework for evaluating and incorporating new experiences and information. It originates and is applied in the mind of knowers. In organisations, it often becomes embedded not only in documents or repositories but also in organisational routines, processes, practices and norms.[14]

Davenport and Prusak go on to emphasise that knowledge cannot be a neat and simple concept. By its very nature it is a mixture of various elements – sometimes it is fluid yet often it is structured, it can be intuitive and hard to capture in words and, above all, knowledge exists within people and is a part of their human complexity and unpredictability. These authors emphasise that although we think of assets as definable and concrete, knowledge assets are much more difficult to pin down.

Therefore this knowledge revolution involves a development that is not necessarily tangible. People could see and touch a 'spinning jenny', or walk into a factory that was being built, but knowledge is far more ephemeral, yet the impact of the knowledge revolution is evident all around us. It has also spawned a vast literature. Some of the literature is conceptual, some is based on the use of information technology, and some has developed into a scientific field of its own where the technocrats appear, Matrix-like, to have taken over.

On a practical level, the two most useful definitions of knowledge management come from the work of Bukowitz and Williams,[15] 'Knowledge management is the process by which the organisation generates wealth from its knowledge or intellectual capital', and Arian Ward,[16] 'It's not about creating an encyclopaedia that captures everything that anybody ever knew. Rather, it's about keeping track of those who know the recipe, and nurturing the culture and the technology that will get them talking.'

The easiest to understand, yet one of the most comprehensive definitions of intellectual capital that I have seen, came from a simple diagram by Stewart in what he called his intellectual capital model.[17] He showed that the total market value of a business is made up of tangible and intangible assets, and that the intangible assets comprise human capital, structural capital (such as patents and networks) and customer capital. This is a simple and helpful description.

Other down-to-earth approaches are available, one of which is the work of Chris Collison and Geoff Parcell in their book *Learning to Fly*.[18] In an entertaining section that shows what they believe to be the difference between *know-why*, *know-how*, *know-what*, *know-who*, *know-where* and *know-when*, they justify their use of the term *knowledge management* to describe the work that they undertake. In an honest and frank assessment of their work they acknowledge that some people have taken issue with them over the use of the term *knowledge management*, as they feel threatened that someone may in a manipulative manner want to control the knowledge they possess, and the two authors accept that it would be quite possible to use terms such as *performance through learning, organisational learning, shared knowledge* or even *working smarter* to describe the work. The appeal of their writing lies in its pragmatic approach and the practical application they have taken in what can be a difficult and esoteric area. Two of their examples are especially attractive and relevant.

The *first example* is based on their belief that knowledge management should become an *unconscious competence* within an organisation, in much the same way as safety and quality campaigners have argued for their disciplines. Their notion of the development of knowledge management is shown as a four-step process from unconscious incompetence to conscious incompetence to conscious competence to unconscious competence. In their *second example* they explain their concept of *peer assist*, which is based on a series of meetings or workshops at which people from different teams are invited to share their insights, experience and knowledge with others. It may be a simple concept, and one that is used in organisations throughout the country, but the captivating attractiveness of their work lies in the set of steps that allows the sharing of knowledge and the creation of new possibilities and actions.

Tacit and explicit knowledge

In most of the writings on knowledge and its management, commentators are careful to distinguish between tacit and explicit knowledge. Leadbeater[19] spends time showing that tacit knowledge is not written down and is difficult to articulate. It is often learned by osmosis and is robust and often intuitive, habitual and reflexive. He contrasts this with explicit knowledge, which he sees as codified, articulated in writing and numbers in books and reports. Thus explicit knowledge, because of the very way in which it is structured, is more transferable than tacit knowledge, and in the transfer from tacit to explicit knowledge, something that is essential for the majority of tacit knowledge to be passed on to someone else, many of the critical nuances may be left out because of its unstructured format. Leadbeater also highlights the emergence of knowledge entrepreneurs who are able to take the commodity of knowledge and make it prosper.

The idea of tacit and explicit knowledge is used imaginatively by Nonaka and Takeuchi[20] to show four basic patterns for creating knowledge at the corporate level within an organisation. Step 1 is *from tacit to tacit*. One individual shares tacit knowledge with another (as with a craftsman and an apprentice) but, because their knowledge never becomes explicit and systematised, it cannot easily be leveraged by the organisation as a whole. Step 2 is *from explicit to explicit*. An expert, such as a finance director, prepares a report for the others on the board to read and understand. The report has synthesised information from many parts of the company, but this process does not really extend the organisation's existing knowledge base either – it merely repositions it. However, when tacit and explicit knowledge interact, Nonaka and Takeuchi show that something powerful happens. Step 3 is *from tacit to explicit*. When someone is able to articulate the foundations of their tacit knowledge and convert it into explicit knowledge, innovative new approaches can be discovered. Step 4 is *from explicit to tacit*. As new explicit knowledge is shared throughout the organisation, other employees begin to internalise it – that is, they use it to broaden, extend and reframe their own tacit knowledge.

This insight from Nonaka and Takeuchi into how knowledge is generated and amassed within the organisation is important and is easier for the lay-person to comprehend than, say, Dixon's[21] work on *the five types of knowledge transfer* (serial/near/far/strategic/expert) or Burton-Jones's[22] *knowledge growth model* of the organisation, although both of these works provide fertile ground for the knowledge management expert. The clear point in all of these approaches is that the knowledge that exists within the healthcare organisation can be managed in much the same way as any other asset.

The utility of tacit and explicit knowledge is also enthrallingly captured in Fahey's[23] topology of knowledge, where she takes a Johari window approach to knowledge to show four dimensions, namely knowledge you know you have, knowledge you know you don't have, knowledge you don't know you have, and knowledge you don't know you don't have. She is to be applauded for this imaginative work.

However, when I have made use of her work with clinicians and managers, I have found it far more productive to take the four domains and to apply them across the fields of knowledge management, intellectual capital, individual and organisational learning and the practice of reflection. Starting with the two negatives in her table first, it is relatively straightforward to define the knowledge that someone does not possess – there are many things someone might be unable to do, such as speaking German or Italian. It is also clear that there are some things that come under the category 'I don't know that I don't know'. This is one of the reasons that constructing opportunities for people to share ideas and to reflect on what has taken place is so very important. I also like to include in this category 'things that I think I know that just aren't so' – this is a particularly important area in dialogue with new entrants to a healthcare organisation, such as non-executive directors, who might believe things about the organisation, possibly based on media coverage, that 'just ain't so'. Fahey's box covering explicit knowledge is correct in its definition (*knowledge that you know you have*), but I am also aware of far too many people who through false modesty, or maybe a general unawareness, are loath to admit to being in possession of explicit knowledge about a particular subject. In these instances the knowledge has to be skilfully drawn out from them. Fahey's quadrant dealing with tacit knowledge has a certain limitation. There are people who actually are well aware of the tacit knowledge they possess, but rather humbly define it as merely something that comes naturally to them. This means that there are times when an individual has to be persuaded, through coaching sessions, that they really are expert in an area even though they may not be conscious of their innate ability. Many people possess first-rate interpersonal, political or social skills and seem oblivious to the fact that others would pay consultants large sums of money to become so well equipped.

TOWARDS NEW WAYS OF THINKING

On many occasions I have started a day by introducing delegates to this nine-dot diagram:

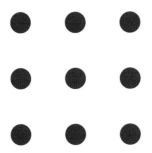

The delegates are asked to join all of the dots using only four straight lines. They are not allowed to take their pens off the paper, they must start at one dot, and each other dot must have a line ending at it or going through it. The delegates are usually bemused, and after much huffing and puffing the vast majority give up, proclaiming that it cannot be done. Inevitably, there are some smug-looking individuals who have achieved the task, and others who having completed the task pretend that they are unable to solve it because their boss, especially if he or she is the trust chief executive, is clearly one of the huffers and puffers.

When the solution is revealed (*see* Figure 4.2) there is a general look of embarrassment as the delegates realise that in their minds they had drawn a box around the nine dots. The exercise is the perfect metaphor to take them into a discussion of the principles of 'thinking outside the box'. In the atmosphere of an away-day it is relatively easy to bring the delegates to a point where they appreciate, and swear allegiance to, the principle of 'thinking outside the box', but back at work it is quite another thing, and they usually revert to type.

The delegates are encouraged to see that all healthcare organisations need radical thinkers – people who are able to think differently, people who are not prepared to utter an automatic 'yes, yes' to the latest idea from the boss, people who are prepared to challenge so-called received wisdom, and people who able to think and contend that there may just be another way of doing things.

I like the doubtless apocryphal story of the boss who encouraged the bright young things in the firm to wear a badge saying, 'Smarter than my boss!' That's the spirit. That's a true recognition that we live in an age where the only competitive advantage, to paraphrase Peter Drucker, is the wisdom of the people we employ. The wise boss encourages such challenging contributions, but far too often those who see the world in a different way, or from a slightly different angle, become ostracised and made to feel unwelcome by their own employer – the cutting remark, the put-down in public, the eyes looking heavenwards at an 'off-the-wall' thought. All of these are designed to ensure conformity to 'the way things are done around here' – the way we have been doing things traditionally despite the changes that are taking place in other healthcare organisations.

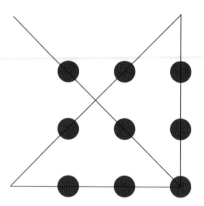

FIGURE 4.2 Nine dots solution

Leaders who think

One of the main reasons why leadership is so difficult is because managers and leaders quite clearly do not know the solutions to many of the problems that they face, and so are presented with a constant stream of new challenges. The comment that 'Leadership would be a safe undertaking if your organisations and communities faced problems for which they already knew the solutions'[24] is a perceptive observation.

So how should healthcare managers respond? I believe that Albert Einstein's well-known observation that 'The significant problems we face cannot be solved at the same level of thinking we were at when we created them'[25] identifies the managerial response which is required. Einstein's challenge is that we need new ways of thinking – thinking that responds to the new challenges of a new age. We need to see organisations becoming places where, to quote Edward de Bono, 'one day dominance by aggression will be replaced by "dominance by wisdom"',[26] an end to what Hamel called 'a world populated by "knowledge workers", [where] there is virtually no time left to think',[27] and people and organisations where 'greenfield minds' are valued more than 'greenfield sites'.[28] Historians continue to judge whether Aneurin Bevan was right when he complained that the 'mediocrity of [Churchill's] thinking is concealed by the majesty of his language',[29] but there are still healthcare organisations whose ability to talk a good game is used to obscure the sparse evidence of their ability to exercise the type of thinking that is needed to respond to the ever-changing circumstances which are being experienced by healthcare organisations at the start of the twenty-first century.

Revolutionary practitioners

The day of the radical thinker has arrived, or at least it should have done. These quotes from a book entitled *Leading the Revolution*[30] describe, in wonderful and typically provocative language, the challenges that organisations should be facing up to in this area:

> There are revolutionaries in your company. But all too often there is no process that lets them be heard. They are isolated and impotent, disconnected from others who share their passions. Their voices are muffled by layers of cautious bureaucrats. They are taught to conform rather than to challenge. And too many senior executives secretly long for a more compliant organisation, rather than a vociferous one.

Imagine how a conservative dad might look upon a kid who comes home with green hair and an eyebrow ring. Well, that's the way top management is likely to view corporate rebels.

> So ask yourself, do you care enough about your integrity to speak the truth and challenge the little lies that jeopardise your company's future? Do you care enough about the future to argue with precedent and stick a thumb in the eye of tradition? . . . Do you care enough about the creative impulse that resides in every human breast that you're ready to help everyone be a revolutionary?

I am not making a case for the 'oddballs' and the 'weirdos' who crop up in all organisations from time to time. They often need to be managed out of the front door, and every healthcare manager should know how to deal with people like that! But I am arguing for the acceptance and active promotion of those people who genuinely see things from a different angle than does the rest of the management team, who are excellent at lateral thinking, who want their team to learn from its successes and failures, who refuse to settle for the status quo, and who believe with a passion that there are better ways of doing things.

At the very least we need people who, to use Burgoyne's taxonomy,[31] are able to move from being merely *effective practitioners* producing *effective practice*, to being practitioners who can develop a theory to support the way they practise, and so become *reflective practitioners* producing *reflective practice*. A reflective practitioner is far more able to teach others and to adapt what is being done to meet the changing circumstances in the workplace. Beyond the *reflective practitioner* there are those who manage to achieve almost Nirvana-like status by producing *critically reflective practice*, and these practitioners, according to Burgoyne, are 'aware that with every practical action they take they are "fixing (temporarily) their belief" and acting on their current best working theory, but they realise that this may also be open to challenge and improvement'.

I know this sounds like academic management-speak, but I assure you that it is not. Rather, it is an acknowledgement that the level of thinking in far too many management activities is just not what it should be. We know from the work of Mintzberg[32] that the *folklore* of management is that 'the manager is a reflective, systematic planner' but that the *fact* is that 'studies show that managers work at an unrelenting pace, that their activities are characterised by brevity, variety and discontinuity – that they are strongly oriented to action and dislike reflective activities'. Or consider the observations of De Bono.[33] Based on his experience of introducing lateral thinking (a phrase and concept that he invented) into an organisation, he notes that the four most harmful attitudes encountered are as follows:
1 apathy ('We have managed all right without it so far')
2 intense enthusiasm ('This is great – this will solve all our problems')
3 know-all ('I have always thought like that anyway')
4 defensive resentment ('It's a new fad that will pass away').

De Bono[34] also shows that thinking can be impaired by four types of complacency, namely comfortable complacency, cosy complacency, arrogant complacency and lack-of-vision complacency.

BOX 4.1 Thirty-one ways to kill an idea

 1 We've tried that one before.
 2 It isn't in the budget (plan!).
 3 We haven't got the staff to do it.
 4 The savings wouldn't come to this division.
 5 Who's going to pay for it?
 6 The intangible risks would be too great.
 7 We're not ready for that yet, but in the fullness of time . . . (let's not rush into things).
 8 That's all very well in theory, but in my experience . . .
 9 This would require the approval of . . . and he will say no!
10 This is the long-term solution . . . We're interested in the here and now.
11 This is the short-term solution . . . We're in this for the long haul.
12 We're already better than our competitors.
13 This is a radical departure from industry practice.

14 You would never get the customer to agree.

15 That's contrary to company policy.

16 But what about the effect on other divisions?

17 We have never done it that way before.

18 It may be okay for XYZ company, but our situation is different.

19 I've been wanting people to do that for a long time, but . . .

20 You can't save half a person.

21 We want our people to think, not just . . .

22 That's not the way we did things at . . .

23 If it's that good, why hasn't somebody tried it before?

24 That's the sort of thing Smith and Jones would do.

25 There are only so many hours in the day.

26 You'll never get that done while ABC is the managing director.

27 Our return on investment is already 39%.

28 Why don't you apply this in XYZ? They really need help.

29 Oh yes, you can prove anything with figures.

30 Yes, that's what he said, but what did he really mean?

31 That's a company problem.

Source: Business Planning Programme, Price Waterhouse[35]

Making space for thinking

Many of the managers, leaders and professionals with whom I have worked will admit, in private conversation, that they find there is very little time in which to think, and that they sometimes feel guilty when they do spend time thinking about their part of the organisation. When was the last time you saw a genuine attempt in your organisation to actively promote thinking time? In contrast, where thinking is a part of normal management practice – and, thank goodness, it is highly valued in many healthcare organisations – there is a belief that the time spent thinking is a crucial part of the success of the particular trust or hospital.

These healthcare organisations devote time to thinking and have available to them a range of techniques to help ensure that their thinking time is highly productive. Each organisation inevitably has its favourite thinking techniques, but two that I have seen used productively are the *six thinking hats*[36] exercise and the concept of *kaleidoscope thinking*.[37]

De Bono's six thinking hats exercise is easy to use, and it is both fun and highly effective in getting people to think differently. By following the book's intro-duction, a facilitator can show that traditional thinking is influenced to a large degree by classical Greek thought based on the famous gang of three – Socrates, Plato and Aristotle. From these roots emerged the basis of verbal Aristotelian logic, in which the whole purpose of their system of thinking was to point out error and to find fault. They believed that if they removed these errors then they would discover the truth. So, concludes de Bono with triumph, finding and pointing out error have been the basis of Western thinking ever since.

Anyone observing the performances of Members of Parliament, or of lawyers in a courtroom, would surely agree with his observation. The main purpose of the exchanges often appears to be the defeat of an opponent's argument rather than the discovery of the best idea or the real reason for a set of circumstances.

The use of de Bono's white, red, black, yellow, green and blue hats to stimulate thinking really does use the experience, intelligence and knowledge of all members of the group, as well as saving time, reducing the role of ego and creating the discipline of observing one facet of an issue at a time. In a humorous manner the approach also enters the managerial vocabulary of an organisation, and I am often told that many weeks after the hats have been used participants in meetings use phrases such as 'If I might be allowed a red hat thought' or 'You will understand that I am talking through my hat at the moment' (my charitable nature assumes that the second comment has something to do with the de Bono exercise!).

Kaleidoscope thinking is not a developed technique in the style of the six thinking hats, and is more an observation by Rosabeth Moss Kanter of practices that are transforming the way in which many firms develop ideas. She shows that:

> Kaleidoscope thinking is a way of constructing new patterns from the fragments of data available – patterns that no one else has imagined because they challenge conventional assumptions about how pieces of the organisation, the marketplace, or the community fit together. A yard sale down the street? So why not a giant yard sale on the Internet? (We call that eBay.) Often it is not reality that is fixed, it is assumptions about reality . . .[37]

Kanter goes on to highlight four organisational practices (with the seductive titles of Monday-morning quarterbacking, expeditions to Labrador, blue sky events and talent shows) that encourage kaleidoscope thinking. The evidence shows that managers catch on to the concept speedily, are willing to participate in the various activities and, most important of all, they see value in undertaking these practices. The various approaches are vehicles that promote thinking in the organisation, and anything that is able to achieve such an outcome should be regarded as worth its weight in gold.

Any objective observer sees clearly that there is a need for organisations – and not just healthcare organisations – to become radical in their pursuit of thinking, to actively promote it, to encourage the so-called corporate rebels, to give an opportunity to young managers as well as to those with grey hair (it is essential to venerate wisdom and experience), and to set aside time in the organisation's hectic schedule for systematic thinking.

THE CHALLENGE FOR MANAGEMENT

In each of the three areas I have set out, namely 'The power of organisational learning', 'Knowledge management and intellectual capital' and 'Towards new ways of thinking', there are numerous clear challenges for healthcare management. In plain and simple language, the challenge is this: 'What are you doing or going to do about it?' A revolution is taking place. A revolution of learning, thinking, knowledge and a new form of capital – intellectual capital – has emerged. To continue with current practices when those practices may well be out of date is not an option for those who want their organisation to thrive. In exceptional cases it may be that the very survival of the organisation will be under threat if changes are not made immediately. There must be an appropriate response from those charged with running the organisation, a response that is geared to taking the organisation forward.

The legendary Peter Drucker in his inimitable way summed it up perfectly. He made the point that all of the productivity gains of the twentieth century could be explained by the work of Frederick Taylor, the father of scientific management, and the improvements that arose as a result of the greater efficiency of employees. Then Drucker, this prophet among management thinkers, added chillingly that 'Work on the productivity of the knowledge worker has barely begun'. That quote deserves to be repeated, and it should be read slowly and deliberately so that the full force of his words can sink in. When Drucker speaks it is worth listening . . . and acting: 'WORK ON THE PRODUCTIVITY OF THE KNOWLEDGE WORKER HAS BARELY BEGUN'.

The challenge I have issued is wider than the role of the knowledge worker, as it concerns the entire knowledge revolution and the crucial role of intellectual capital within a healthcare organisation. Imagine the farmer of centuries ago, who ignored or perhaps even scorned the discoveries and advances made by Townsend, Coke, Tull and others like them. What would have happened to those farmers? The answer seems to be straightforward – they would have been left behind with primitive methods to farm the land. What of those people who dismissed the efforts of Watt, Hargreaves, Crompton, Arkwright and the like? What became of them? They would have been sidelined – an economic irrelevancy as the economy boomed and the economic and social landscape became transformed.

Without any doubt most organisations around the world have realised that they need to respond to this new revolution, and so have put in place the necessary structures and systems to capitalise on the advances that can be made. However, there are others who are slow to respond or who have not realised the full extent of the revolution that is taking place. In the very week that I wrote these words, in the first half of 2004, I met the research director of a mega-million-pound, well-known public-sector organisation who said 'I haven't got my mind around this intellectual capital thing yet'. I was too polite, or perhaps too cowardly, to utter the '*What?!*' that was my immediate response. Into my mind came a picture of a farmer who was blissfully ignorant of the latest Townsend development, and a small clothing manufacturer who was unaware that Hargreaves and others were about to revolutionise their world. In those days – an age without the benefit of technological communication – the lack of appreciation was far more understandable. However, in this day and age – a time when communication is both global and instant – there can be little excuse for those who are unaware that the third revolution is taking place all around them.

At the very least, healthcare organisations should implement the four-step process for managing intellectual capital advocated by Stewart,[38] which is briefly illustrated by the following four headings. Organisations need to (i) identify and evaluate the role of knowledge in the organisation; (ii) match the revenues found with the knowledge assets that produce them; (iii) develop strategies to invest in and explore intellectual assets; and (iv) improve the efficiency of knowledge work.

Often these precious assets (the people and the intellectual capital that they produce) are not properly managed. They are treated as easily dispensable resources, managed in ways which suggest that they are equipment on an assembly line rather than the very lifeblood of the future organisation, and they are not given the space to think about and experiment with new ways of working. The knowledge that they possess is not garnered as intellectual capital, the 'left hand' in many instances does not know what the 'right hand' is doing, and the methods of developing the capacity of the scarce and precious knowledge worker leave much to be desired. This is one of the reasons why so many people leave their employers and set up their own business, which then develops and sometimes even threatens the survival of the original parent organisation. If only the 'parent' had seen the potential in their former employees – and now rivals. Wise healthcare organisations recognise the potential of new ideas and provide their staff with the scope to grow and prosper, even if this is under the 'parent's' sensitive direction.

Key actions

1 To develop your understanding of organisational learning you should obtain a copy of Peter Senge's *Fifth Discipline*, read at the very least the first 40–50 pages of the book, and then talk to colleagues who share your belief in the importance of organisational learning.

2 The concept of intellectual capital and its three main components – social, organisational and human capital – is becoming an increasingly important issue. To what extent have you and your organisation taken account of this?

3 I realise that there are pressures on you to deliver key objectives, but you really should set aside time to encourage meaningful thinking and personal reflection.

REFERENCES

1 Stewart TA (1998) *Intellectual Capital*. Nicholas Brealey, London.
2 Beckhard R (1997) Who needs us? In: DF Van Eynde, *et al.* (eds) *Organization Development Classics*. Jossey-Bass, San Francisco, CA.
3 Stewart TA (1998) *Intellectual Capital*. Nicholas Brealey, London.
4 Senge PM (1990) *The Fifth Discipline: the art and practice of the learning organization*. Century Business, London.
5 Mumford A and Gold J (2004) *Management Development: strategies for action*. Chartered Institute of Personnel and Development, London.
6 Garvin DA (2003) *Learning in Action*. Harvard Business School Press, Boston, MA.
7 Beckhard R and Pritchard W (1992) *Changing the Essence: the art of creating and leading*

fundamental change in organisations. Jossey-Bass, San Francisco, CA, and John Wiley and Sons, New York.

8 Senge PM (1990) *The Fifth Discipline: the art and practice of the learning organization.* Century Business, London.

9 Senge PM (1990) The leader's new work: building learning organizations. *Sloan Management Review,* 32: 7–22.

10 Grint K (1996) The non-learning and learning organisation. In: B Garratt (ed.) *The Fish Rots from the Head.* HarperCollins Business, London.

11 Mayo A and Lank E (1994) *The Power of Learning.* Chartered Institute of Personnel and Development, London.

12 de Geus A (1997) *The Living Company: growth, learning and longevity in business.* Nicholas Brealey, London.

13 My recollection of these characters from the agricultural and industrial revolutions has been refreshed by the wonderful *Children's Britannica,* and some of the words I use are from its text. *Children's Britannica* (1991) Encyclopaedia Britannica, London.

14 Davenport TH and Prusak L (1998) *Working Knowledge: how organisations manage what they know.* Harvard Business School Press, Boston, MA.

15 Bukowitz WR and Williams RL (1999) *The Knowledge Management Fieldbook.* Pearson Education, London.

16 Arian Ward of Work Frontiers International. Quoted in: Collison C and Parcell G (2001) *Learning to Fly: practical lessons from one of the world's leading knowledge companies.* Capstone, Oxford.

17 Stewart TA (1998) *Intellectual Capital.* Nicholas Brealey, London.

18 Collison C and Parcell G (2001) *Learning to Fly: practical lessons from one of the world's leading knowledge companies.* Capstone, Oxford.

19 Leadbeater C (2000) *Living on Thin Air.* Penguin, Harmondsworth.

20 Nonaka I and Takeuchi H (1995) *The Knowledge-Creating Company.* Oxford University Press, Oxford.

21 Dixon NM (2000) *Common Knowledge.* Harvard Business School Press, Boston, MA.

22 Burton-Jones A (2001) *Knowledge Capitalism.* Oxford University Press, Oxford.

23 The model developed by Liam Fahey of Babson College is included in: Stewart TA (1998) *Intellectual Capital.* Nicholas Brealey, London.

24 Heifetz RA and Linsky M (2002) *Leadership on the Line.* Harvard Business School Press, Boston, MA.

25 Covey SR (1989) *The Seven Habits of Highly Effective People.* Simon and Schuster, London.

26 de Bono E (2000) *New Thinking for the New Millennium.* Penguin, Harmondsworth.

27 Hamel G (2000) *Leading the Revolution.* Harvard Business School Press, Boston, MA.

28 Wickens PD (1995) *The Ascendant Organisation.* Palgrave Macmillan, Basingstoke.

29 Shea M (1994) *Personal Impact: the art of good communication.* Mandarin, London.

30 Hamel G (2000) *Leading the Revolution.* Harvard Business School Press, Boston, MA.

31 Burgoyne J and Reynolds M (eds) (1977) *Management Learning: integrating perspectives in theory and practice.* Sage, London.

32 Mintzberg H (1973) *The Nature of Managerial Work.* Longman, New York.

33 de Bono E (1990) *Lateral Thinking for Management.* Penguin, Harmondsworth.

34 de Bono E (1992) *Sur/Petition.* Fontana, London.

35 These points were given to me as a handout many years ago by a Price Waterhouse consultant at a business planning training event.

36 de Bono E (2000) *Six Thinking Hats*®. Penguin, Harmondsworth.

37 Kanter RM (2001) *e.volve: succeeding in the digital world of tomorrow*. Harvard Business School Press, Boston, MA.

38 Stewart TA (2001) The intellectual capital model. In: *The Wealth of Knowledge*. Nicholas Brealey, London.

CHAPTER 5

Human resource management

PRELUDE

For over 30 years I have been associated with the world of personnel and human resource (HR) management. In the 1970s, the dominating influence for me was the world of industrial relations, and it appeared that every day brought new challenges to be resolved. In the 1980s, the focus became development and the management of change. In the 1990s, it centred around strategic HR, leadership and organisation development, and more recently my emphasis has been on linking academic concepts of HR management with its practical application. Throughout that time, and no matter what the particular personnel emphasis, the profession of HR management has seemed to be on a constant mission to justify its own existence and its role in the organisational hierarchy. Why should that be?

As I prepared to write this chapter I spent a considerable amount of time reading the work of leading UK and US academics on various aspects of HR management (some of the authors are cited, others are not), and I read just about every recent publication from the Chartered Institute of Personnel and Development. In addition, I spoke to many people, joined a UK forum that hosts executive seminars with leading international HR thinkers, and thought in some depth about my own journey through personnel and HR management. As a result I have come to some conclusions that will serve as propositions to underpin what I have to say throughout this chapter. They are stated boldly or, perhaps in some people's eyes, rather presumptuously. Nevertheless, they are as follows:

➤ I believe HR management to be a noble activity because it links itself with the importance and dignity of people and commits itself to bringing the very best out of those people

➤ I believe that first-class HR practices make a direct, relevant and substantial contribution to the 'bottom-line' performance of the healthcare organisation, and to all other types of organisation

➤ I believe that the key determinant of effectiveness and relevance in the HR function is the quality of its own professional staff.

I did warn you – three bold assertions based on the academic and applied HR literature, discussions with leading thinkers in the HR field, and three decades of being closely and sometimes less closely associated with the profession.

INTRODUCTION

Imagine that you are about to be appointed to a key HR job by the chief executive of one of two organisations.

The first chief executive – or managing director (MD) as he calls himself – is the owner of a small business, one of the Small to Medium Enterprises (SMEs) that are the very backbone of the UK economy. As the business begins to prosper, and the number of staff employed increases, the MD decides, after hearing the advice of a business expert at one of the local small business seminars, to hire for the first time ever an HR specialist. After placing an advertisement and holding some interviews, the 'very person' is found, someone who fills the MD with confidence that this new HR manager will help to improve the business even further. In the first meeting with the HR expert, the MD decides that there is a need to explain the main priorities of the business in greater detail than was possible at the interview – the type of business environment, the profitability and growth expectations for the next five years, the types of product and service that are sold and the range of markets are explained. When the MD is certain that the HR manager has a basic grasp of these key facts, he explains, again in more detail than was possible at the interview, that the HR job involves looking after the people side of the business. This means being responsible for hiring the right type of staff, making sure that they are properly trained for the jobs they will be doing, devising a payment-by-results scheme and getting it agreed by everyone concerned, looking after the legal and personnel administration procedures (including health and safety), making sure that the employees are happy with their lot so that there is a 'good feel in the air', and above all making sure that all HR activities are undertaken with one eye on the profitability of the business, because without continuing profit there will be no business in the long term. In this business, explains the MD, the long term can be a matter of 9–12 months if profitability is not kept at the top of the list of priorities. Finally, the MD wishes the HR manager the best of luck and offers them advice and support on any issue at any time.

Although these circumstances are imaginary, and somewhat elementary, nevertheless it is the case that every day of the week this very scenario is being played out in small businesses across the country. It may be that the MD does not go out and recruit an HR specialist. It may be that one of the partners or managers takes responsibility for the HR activities, but the general principles of what I have described are taking place, and they are taking place in the demanding world where profit and loss are key elements in the short term. This is no academic or long-term strategic exercise for these businesses – it is concerned with the very stuff of business survival, and if they get it wrong they could go under.

The second chief executive is the head of a large, well-known, teaching NHS trust with clinical services that have a thoroughly deserved high reputation across the country. The chief executive has just appointed a new HR director to the main board. Although the conversation between the chief executive and the HR director is more sophisticated, the number of employees far greater, the issues more complicated and the 'balance sheet' more impressive, I would contend that the substance of the conversations between the owner of the SME and the first-time HR manager, and between the chief executive and the HR director of the large NHS trust, will be identical in essence. The figures may be different, and the language more fanciful in the trust, but the two jobs have a striking similarity – the two HR employees are there to look after the people side of their respective organisations, from hiring staff to developing them and getting the best out of them, and they have to do it in a way which makes sure that the 'bottom-line' requirements and the future needs of the organisations are met.

I recognise that the HR manager from the SME would not be able to undertake the NHS job. The difference in scale and the complexity inherent in it would overwhelm an inexperienced newcomer, or one better suited to small companies. However, the point I am making, and will continue to make, is that although there are clear differences of scale and complexity between the jobs, the very essence of their work is similar. The single-handed HR specialist knows what the SME owner wants and what has to be done to contribute to the business. What is more, the owner also knows what is needed from the HR person, and will be able to decide (admittedly rather crudely and potentially erroneously, if based solely on the question of profit) whether the HR manager is delivering the goods and represents a wise investment. In the larger NHS organisation there should be little difference. Large organisations should know what is needed from their HR people, and they should know what is being delivered, but the evidence suggests that in many large organisations, and perhaps in some NHS trusts, there is a lack of clarity about what has to be delivered and also how it influences the 'bottom line' of the organisation. It is this very lack of clarity – something that has beset the world of personnel and HR since almost the start of the last century – which has resulted in complex attempts to demonstrate the worthwhileness of something that should be self-evident – HR is beneficial to the 'bottom line' of the organisation. This lack of clarity is puzzling – if an organisation does not believe that employing a specialist to look after the extremely important resource of people is a very wise investment, then there are two very pertinent questions to ask. Why on earth were the HR managers and directors employed in the first place? And why do organisations continue to spend scarce resources on the HR function? An organisation either believes in the function, on the basis of hard evidence, or it does not.

HR MANAGEMENT AND THE 'BOTTOM LINE'

I can understand the pressures on an SME taking a first-time decision to employ an HR professional, and the newly appointed HR person trying as hard as possible to show the connection between HR activity and the performance of the business. What I find hard to understand is the on-going tussle in large organisations to show that the HR function is a worthwhile activity. I believe passionately in the need for organisations above a certain size to have a professional HR function, so I remain perplexed at the way in which so many of these organisations appear to agonise over what appears to me to be a self-evident truth – professional HR departments are good for the health of the organisation and the people employed in them. If chief executives do not believe that to be the case then again I ask why the HR people were appointed in the first place, and also why HR directors lack the confidence and ability to demonstrate to their peers and bosses that they are as important as the marketing function or the finance professionals. As I shall show in the next section and later, academics claim that they are now able to *prove* that there is a direct link between the HR function and 'bottom-line' performance, and yet far too often HR directors still suffer from a reticence about the value of the corporate functions that they lead. Why should this be? The answer to this difficult and frequently asked question must surely be found in the origins of the profession and in the type of HR professionals an organisation employs.

HEALTHCARE'S 'BOTTOM LINE'

Within healthcare, the work of Michael A West and his colleagues[1] to demonstrate the link between the management of employees and patient mortality in acute hospitals has received considerable prominence. West, *et al.* recognised that a substantial amount of organisational behaviour research had examined the impact of HR management on organisational outcomes but that little research had been undertaken to explore this relationship in hospital settings.

Their research was 'designed to determine whether there are links between HRM practices and hospital performance as indicated by patient mortality data' and importantly they set out to determine which HR practices affect quality of care and effectiveness:

> . . . to determine whether there are links between HRM practices and hospital performance as indicated by patient mortality data. The aim was to show not just whether there is a link between human resource management practices, quality of care and effectiveness, but which practices affect these outcomes.[2]

Although the researchers list certain cautions concerning their findings – such as the small sample size, the fact that 'the sample size varies between analyses', and the mortality variables being from different timescales – nevertheless they are confident to declare

> [t]his study revealed a significant association between the management of employees in acute hospitals and the levels of patient mortality within those hospitals . . . Specifically, the sophistication and extensiveness of appraisal and training for hospital employees and the percentage of staff working in teams in the hospitals were all significantly associated with measures of patient mortality.[3]

To possess research showing 'strong links between HR practices and patient mortality in hospitals' and to be able to present evidence that it may be possible to 'influence hospital performance significantly by implementing sophisticated and extensive training and appraisal systems, and encouraging a high percentage of employees to work in teams' should be a boon to healthcare HR managers. My understanding is that some have used this research effectively and others, for reasons I discuss later, are practically unaware of the importance of linking practice to the 'bottom line'.

Recently, I included reference to this research in a report I had been commissioned to prepare on an aspect of HR development – the client asked me to delete reference to West's work as the eventual recipient of the report had such an antipathy to HRM that my inclusion of this reference would be counter-productive to acceptance of my report's full recommendations. (The problem was HRM and not Michael West, I hasten to add.) Human resource management may be essential but in some healthcare locations it has much to do to prove its effectiveness.

STAND UP AND BE COUNTED

As I read the appointment section in the Sunday newspapers and professional journals I see a constant stream of advertisements for HR people who are required to help transform a particular organisation, and often these are public-sector appointments. It seems that every medium to large-scale organisation goes to great lengths to recruit the best HR person it can find. Yet there remains this ambivalence about whether or not HR's contribution to the performance of the organisation is valued or not. Why are the HR professionals so unsure of their worth? Why are they reluctant to get on the front foot and declare aloud that HR people are in the business of developing people, who for the vast majority of organisations represent their most important asset? HR practitioners need to shout aloud that they are not engaged in HR jobs because they could not get a job in any other function, but they are employed in HR management because they are expert at what they do and they believe, with a passion, that what they do is extremely important to the health of the organisation.

I believe that one of the reasons for this lack of assertiveness is that many HR directors know that some of their people are not up to scratch. It may be true that they would find it hard to get a job in another activity, or they may be passive individuals who are unsure about their true role in the organisation, or they may be like the apocryphal welfare officer who started work in the 1960s and, without moving office or changing his responsibilities, became a industrial relations officer in the 1970s, an employee relations officer in the 1980s, and in the 1990s, and just before he retired in 2000, an HR officer. He didn't change – it was just the name plaque on his door that was unscrewed and replaced every few years! I know I exaggerate to make the point, but there are too many of these individuals, whom I have met in some organisations and sectors more than in others, who cannot pass muster. Fortunately, the opposite is also true, and in those organisations where the HR function is staffed by bright, able, committed and talented people there is seldom a heart-searching debate about the meaning of HR management and its contribution to corporate life – they know that they are vibrant and making a positive contribution. I can remember when the personnel supremo, Sir Len Peach, lent his considerable influence and weight to the infant Personnel Standards Lead Body, and they issued a statement exhorting that to be effective in personnel three criteria had to be met:

1 the practitioner had to be technically competent in both advice given and actions taken
2 all personnel activities had to be related to the performance of the organisation
3 the personnel practitioner had to be accepted by senior colleagues as 'one of us' on a personal basis as well as on the basis of the role held.

These are wise words, and they are as relevant today as they were in the early 1990s. It is essential that they are put into practice by everyone.

BOX 5.1 Five types of poor personnel/HR practitioner: a dying breed?

1 *The welfare type*: a pleasing personality ('hail fellow well met') who is wonderful at visiting the sick (but not at controlling absence), who does a first-class schools presentation on behalf of the organisation (but makes little contribution to recruitment strategy and practice), who may run a mile when the going gets tough, and who possesses the longest list of trite sayings and jargon you have ever heard.
2 *The reject*: everyone knows that this person was 'dumped' on the personnel department because they could no longer cut it as a line manager. What is more, no other department wanted them, and they could not be sacked for some complex legal reason, so the personnel department was the obvious new employer. Personnel were pleased to receive them as they came as a 'free good' with the salary cost hidden in some corporate overhead. A variation on this theme is the ex-trade union shop steward who did a good job representing members but who has been subsequently rejected and needs to be found a new post and department.
3 *The trouble raiser*: the preferred sobriquet would be 'trouble shooter', but every-one knows that wherever this person goes there is trouble. They relish it, thrive on it and for some extraordinary reason actually fan the flames of discontent instead of extinguishing them. As far as this person is concerned, the halcyon days were the 1970s when there was an industrial relations fire starting or raging in almost every part of the organisation.
4 *The mountaineer*: this person can create mountains out of molehills. Apparently simple, straightforward management tasks are turned into complex issues requiring meetings that become committees, working groups that require project plans, and reams of paper from which it is likely that strategies will emerge. They cannot just get on and solve a problem – they have to tackle it in a way that beggars belief.
5 *The rule keeper*: every procedure, condition of employment, regulation, em-ployment law and European convention can be recited by heart and with a relish to explain the three best reasons why something the organisation needs to do for the prosperity of the organisation and its people is against the law, probably a code of practice and some other fundamental principle. The organisation actually wants to keep the law and conform to best practice – what

is galling about this person is the relish with which the hindrances are pointed out and the sense that being a barrier, rather than a bridge, is something which the person actually enjoys.

HR SOFTIES?

A second and frequently cited reason for the questioning of HR management is the temptation for the function to be associated with what are seen to be the 'soft' issues of the organisation, and the reluctance to get involved in those issues that resemble trench warfare. It was one of the strengths of the industrial relations phase of personnel that it was seen to earn its spurs by getting into the heat of the battle and fighting for the survival of the organisation. One of the ironies, of course, is that this turbulence enhanced the standing of the function, and there was more than one industrial relations manager who regretted the passing of the days of struggle, as this coincided with a diminution in the influence of industrial relations practitioners. The HR practitioner must show that whether they are dealing with 'soft' or 'hard' issues, the 'human' part of the job or the 'resources' part of it, they are able and willing to act expertly with the needs of the organisation at the forefront of their actions.

VICTIMS OF HISTORY?

Thirdly, even the origins of the function can present a reason for the difficulty that the profession sometimes has in asserting itself. There cannot be anyone alive today who remembers the earliest days when personnel was a welfare activity supporting the social and humanitarian activities of enlightened employers at the turn of the twentieth century. However, there are many people alive, and some who are still in employment, who can remember the personnel function as little more than an administrative service. Karen Legge, in her excellent book *Human Resource Management*, traces the roots of personnel and examines the four models (normative, descriptive-functional, critical-evaluative and descriptive-behavioural) of personnel management, and in quoting the then Institute of Personnel Management classic definition of what its members actually practised demonstrates the seeming lack of dynamism of the profession at that time:

> 'Personnel management is a responsibility of all those who manage people, as well as being a description of the work of those who are employed as specialists. It is that part of management which is concerned with people at work and with their relationships within an enterprise . . .'[4]

No wonder so many people saw personnel, in the words of US academics Ritzer and Trice,[5] as reacting to problems, being passive, defending the status quo, not helping to shape management thinking, not being a risk taker, not being business oriented and operating in a vacuum.

The arrival of HR management should have heralded a new dawn. Although there are numerous books that explain, usually from an academic perspective, the differences between personnel and the HR function, for most of the people I have worked with the favourite way of explaining the difference is Storey's well-known chart,[6] which can be found in most HR textbooks. Storey identifies 27 dimensions of personnel and HR management, under the sub-headings of beliefs and assumptions, strategic aspects, line management and key levers, and shows how the HR function differs significantly from personnel.

Here lies the challenge for all personnel practitioners, and especially those who are called HR managers but who know, in their heart of hearts, that they are performing old-fashioned personnel roles. The challenge lies in how one acts, what values drive the action and the extent to which the HR or personnel professional is an accepted part of the top management team and contributes to the 'bottom line' of the healthcare organisation. The title someone uses is not the key issue – after all, the professional body for HR professionals still retains the title 'personnel' rather than 'HR'.

HOW THE HR/PERSONNEL PROFESSIONAL SHOULD ACT

It is time I stopped this general hectoring and suggested the seven ways in which I believe an HR professional should demonstrate competence and add value to a healthcare organisation.

1 Recognise and value the dignity of people

At the start of this chapter I explained that my thoughts on the HR function would be governed by three key propositions. One of these was that *I believe HR management to be a noble activity because it links itself with the importance and dignity of people and commits itself to bringing the very best out of those people.* This belief underpins my first recommendation on how HR professionals should approach their work.

Anyone who has read the Universal Declaration of Human Rights must be emotionally affected by the principles contained in the Declaration, and by the fact that there are countries in the world where these basic human rights are being flagrantly ignored. I realise that the Declaration is predominantly an attempt to deter countries, their leaders and people from indulging in atrocities that have 'outraged the conscience of mankind', to quote the Declaration. However, I think it is also possible to read the Declaration through the lens of employment practice – HR professionals claim that people are the most important resource in an organisation, and that HR professionals are in the 'people business'. If that is the case, there are some fundamental questions to be asked. How do your employment practices square with the basic requirements in the Declaration? Are your people treated with the dignity that they deserve? Are you the custodian of the corporate conscience on these matters? And if you are not, then who is?

Here are some quotes from the Declaration that I consider to be relevant to the practice of HR.

- Recognition of the inherent dignity and of the equal and inalienable rights of all members of the human family . . .
- . . . human rights should be protected by the rule of law.
- . . . faith in . . . the dignity and growth of the human person and in the equal rights of men and women . . .
- No one shall be subjected to arbitrary . . . attacks upon his honour or reputation . . .
- Everyone has the right to freedom of opinions without interference . . .
- No one may be compelled to belong to an association.
- Everyone has the right to work . . .
- Everyone . . . has the right to equal pay for equal work.
- Everyone has the right . . . to join trade unions
- Everyone has the right to rest and leisure . . .
- Everyone has the right to a standard of living adequate for the health and well-being of himself and his family . . .
- Motherhood and childhood are entitled to special care and assistance . . .

Some may think that I am going soft in my old age! I assure you that this is not the case. I recognise that some parts of the Declaration are 'aspirational' rather than absolute rights when it comes to the world of employment, but I contend that the points itemised above are basic human rights and that any organisation should see it to be a part of their role in society, wherever possible, to uphold them. HR professionals should see them as issues to underpin the development of policies, and as the *raison d'être* for so much of what passes as HR practice. Before you decide that my 'soft' approach is unreasonable, let me respond by readily acknowledging that there is a 'hard' side to the HR function, just as there is a difference between the 'human' and the 'resource' side of the work of the profession (more about this later). Although I accept the 'hard' side of HR, I also contend that there is a need for HR professionals to state their beliefs about people, and to act on those beliefs, rather than merely chanting the mantra about people being 'our most important asset'. Prove it. Show it. Invest in people. If you really believe it to be the case that people are your most important asset, then my challenge to you – and I admit that this is mainly a moral challenge – is to be an HR professional who:

➤ has a deep-seated belief in the dignity of people
➤ ensures that people are treated properly, even when tough management decisions which affect their current and future employment are being taken
➤ regards the principle of how people are treated as a moral issue and as one that, in both the short and long term, benefits the reputation and thereby the overall health of the organisation.

This belief in a principle affects both *what* you do and *how* you do it. You may have to make someone redundant, or dismiss an employee on the grounds of capability or conduct, but you can still act with a regard for their basic human dignity. We should also remember that it is quite possible to be very successful in a healthcare organisation, to get promoted beyond one's wildest dreams, and still feel that the basic need to be treated with dignity is not being observed. I have seen enough employee attitude surveys to know this to be true. HR professionals are concerned with human beings, not inanimate resources, and those people need to be treated as such.

2 Assert the importance and value of the HR function to your healthcare organisation

The Chartered Institute of Personnel and Development issued two research reports that constitute some of the most important personnel/HR publications I have ever read, and this research substantiates my second proposition – *that first-class HR practices make a direct, relevant and substantial contribution to the 'bottom-line' performance of the healthcare organisation, and to all other types of organisation.*

The first report is *Effective People Management,*[7] based on research among 610 managers responsible for the HR function and 462 CEOs, across 835 organisations in the UK. Although it found that 'most managers only pay lip service to the idea that people are their most important assets' and that 'there is clearly considerable scope in British industry to improve HRM', the research shows that 'the effective use of a wide range of progressive HR practices is linked to superior performance'. This finding, according to the reputable team of researchers, is in addition to the 'large and growing body of evidence that demonstrates a wholly positive relationship between people management and development practice and organisational performance'. HR managers should be jumping up and down with joy – what they have always believed has been supported by reputable research. But why is it that I fear many HR managers do not realise that the research is available, and even if they are aware of its existence they are probably too reticent about shouting it from their headquarters' rooftops? That is why the researchers can state confidently that 'it is evident that the message is still not getting through to certain sections of the business community' and that 'personnel specialists need to be more positive about developing measures to value the human contribution'. This is a highly significant finding. Here is objective evidence that the work of the HR function, when applied professionally and appropriately, adds value to the organisation, including healthcare organisations. Sing it out loud, personnel and HR professionals!

The second research report is entitled *Understanding the People and Performance Link: unlocking the black box.* The report recognises that previous studies have shown the connection between effective HR practices and organisational performance, but highlights the fact that:

> none has explained the nature of this connection – in other words, how and why HR practices impact on performance. This is commonly referred to as the 'black box' problem, and the main purpose of our study was to unlock the 'black box' to show the way in which HR practices . . . impact on performance.[8]

In their study, researchers from the University of Bath show the importance of an organisation having what they call a 'big idea' – a clear mission underpinned by values – and of that big idea being embedded, connected, enduring, collective and 'measured and managed' within the culture of the organisation. They also demonstrate the significant role of line management in making the HR practices effective, and in a report containing abundant wise counsel they add sound advice that will resonate with experienced personnel practitioners: 'getting existing policies to work better is more likely to pay dividends in terms of increasing commitment than developing new policies'. They go on to show the ways in which the practice of the HR function can make a positive and valuable contribution.

To attempt to précis the report in a few short paragraphs would be to do it a grave injustice, and in any case that is not my purpose in quoting from it. My point is that these extremely important reports, along with others, such as the work of Michael West, *et al.* (*see* page 92) should give HR managers enough ammunition to be able to proclaim to their management and clinical colleagues that hard evidence exists to demonstrate the contribution made by the HR function to the success of the organisation. HR professionals should learn large chunks of the text of these reports 'off by heart' and recite them loudly to colleagues who express agnosticism about the value of the personnel endeavour.

3 Demonstrate how the HR function is contributing to the 'bottom line'

Having established the general principle that the HR function does benefit the organisation, there has never been a better time to introduce some set of measures to demonstrate the people contribution that is being made to the 'bottom-line' performance of the healthcare organisation.

Most organisations recognise the utility of what has been called *intellectual capital* (*see* Chapter 4). They recognise that the days of calculating capital, the typical worth of an organisation, merely on the basis of traditional assets such as land and buildings has serious limitations, and that there is a need to account for the intellectual capital of the enterprise. Some in the private sector argue, rather simplistically in my view, that if one takes the market value of an organisation and subtracts from that the balance-sheet value of the business, then the difference is the organisation's intellectual capital. The debate over the legitimacy of the precise calculations need not bother us. It is the principle at the heart of definition, and the very existence of the notion of intellectual capital, that needs to be grasped at this juncture.

The intellectual capital in the organisation is usually seen as having three components:
1 the knowledge held within the organisation (and usually not tapped to its full potential); this is where knowledge management gurus can be very helpful
2 the capital that arises through the contacts which the organisation, and the individuals within it, have with other organisations and people
3 the human capital – the skills, knowledge and experience of its people (its most valuable resource, if one believes the rhetoric).

Human capital is defined by the OECD[9] as 'the knowledge that individuals acquire during their life and use to produce goods, services or ideas in market or non-market circumstances'. A more current and popular definition within the world of HR experts comes from Bontis:

> Human capital represents the human factor in the organisation; the combined intelligence, skills and expertise that gives the organisation its distinctive character. The human elements of the organisation are those that are capable of learning, changing, innovating and providing the creative thrust which if properly motivated can ensure the long-term survival of the organisation.[10]

Scarbrough and Elias[11] have written a valuable guide on the theory and practice of human capital. The first half of their work examines the extensive body of literature on human capital, and the second part reviews the experiences of 10 organisations 'making real and deliberate efforts to better understand the contribution of their people to the success of their organisation'. In their review of the literature they make the telling point that:

> Given the sophistication of modern management techniques, it seems curious, to say the least, that there should still be a question mark over managers' ability to adequately understand, value and deploy what so many experts agree is one of their major sources of competitive advantage, namely their people. If organisations were as backward in identifying and reporting on any of the other major resources at their command, it would be viewed as nothing short of scandalous.

The case studies are based on Marks and Spencer, Tesco, Xerox, Norwich Union Insurance, Motorola, Shell UK, BT, BAE Systems, an automobile manufacturer and an investment bank. The case study experiences make fascinating reading, as does the authors' observation that 'none of the case study firms explicitly used the term "human capital". Indeed, we found some resistance to the term on the grounds that it reduced individual employees to the status of economic units'.[12] Common sense prevails, it seems. These organisations realise that employees are people, not capital.

BOX 5.2 Human capital: our greatest resource

Imagine if someone told you that it was possible to improve the return on your organisation's most important assets by as much as 10–20%. How would you respond? Would you show interest and want to find out more? Or would you be cynical and question the motives of the individual? Would you think it was a con trick, or classify it as another of those management fads that promised the world and usually made little difference?

More and more managers are realising that it is possible to improve the return on the organisation's most important assets by at least 10%. The assets in question, of course, are the people of the organisation – the staff, the human resource, the human capital (to use the in-vogue term). Board directors, and not just HR professionals, are realising that an organisation's staff really are its most important resource, and that the all-too-familiar comment in the annual report, 'our staff are our greatest asset', might just be true. And they are beginning to understand that the contribution their people make can help to transform the performance of their organisation.

A case of neglect?

Eight or nine years ago I read of a US management consultant who claimed that when he asked the employees of his clients how much of their talent was being used by their employers, the answer he usually got was 'about 50%'. Quite frankly, I did not believe the figures, and decided to ask a similar question of healthcare and public-sector conference delegates when I spoke at their seminars. I asked them 'How much of your available and appropriate ability is used by your organisation?'. (I was always careful to explain what I meant by the words: 'available' meant what they were prepared to give to their organisation, so it took into account work–life balance issues; 'appropriate' meant that the organisation needed them to give it; 'ability' meant the talent, skills, knowledge or competence that they possessed; 'how much' was a request for a percentage figure.) I discussed the notions behind the question, and to my very great surprise I started to obtain similar answers. The average figure was between 50% and 60%, and the range of responses was usually between 30% and 80%. (I readily acknowledge that this survey has a number of statistical limitations, including the numbers surveyed and in terms of validity.) When I explained my findings to some senior managers of a well-known organisation they were not particularly surprised and explained that they spent a large part of their time 'wading through treacle' – in other words, fighting the bureaucracy that seemed to militate against them giving their best performance.

I have related these facts to many people, from all walks of life, and typically I am greeted with a nod of the head, a shrug of the shoulders and a smile of resignation. It may be that my friends and colleagues are being kind to me, but the impression I get is that they are not particularly surprised. It squares with their experience of life. One such colleague and friend is John Noble, the director of the Greenleaf Centre for Servant-Leadership UK. He told me that he had heard Sir John Harvey-Jones say something similar many years before. John had been in the audience at University College London in 1994 when Harvey-Jones was launching his book *All Together Now*. During the question-and-answer session, someone asked Sir John, 'How much of the talent of our workforce do we use?', and Harvey-Jones immediately responded '40%'. It may not have been an answer backed up by research, but it was a figure from his heart, and it demonstrated his belief that organisations often under-utilise the talent on offer to them.

Surely things have improved since 1994? Quite recently, a client told me about an employee opinion survey she had commissioned. Her board wanted to find out what its employees thought about aspects of life in their organisation, so they commissioned the internationally recognised opinion research company ORC International to conduct the survey and to compare her organisation's results with their database of 1.1 million employees in 150 other organisations. The responses to Question 38 of the survey, 'How satisfied are you with the training you received for your present job?', were most revealing. It showed that only 57% on average were satisfied and that the responses ranged from 32–81%. I was astonished when I realised the significance of their figures for the 30–80% I had found in my 'statistically challenged' surveys.

I know their question was not the same as mine, and that you would be justified in claiming that I am not comparing 'apples with apples' in a precise academic style. I plead guilty to this, but I want to present further circumstantial evidence to make what I consider to be an overwhelming case.

The issue of capability

If you are a fan of BBC2's *Newsnight* programme then you will know that there are times when Jeremy Paxman finds it hard to contain a contemptuous sneer for the intellectual inadequacies of the person he is interviewing. When he interviewed Professor Michael Porter, from the Institute of Competitiveness at Harvard Business School, Paxman was clearly in awe of him. Porter is an intellectual giant and was commissioned by the Department of Trade and Industry and the Economic and Social Research Council to investigate the current state of UK competitiveness.

Porter's report 'demonstrates the UK's strengths in terms of science and engineering, its supportive market framework, and its improved macro-economic environment . . . [but] . . . highlights continued weaknesses in terms of skills, clusters of interconnected companies and innovation'. His view is supported by the 2002 Global Competitiveness Report (GCR), which praises the UK for being open to international trade and investment, for having very low regulatory barriers to competition, and for its sophisticated capital markets, but criticises it for 'skills deficits in the labour force despite favourable international rankings on educational achievement'.

The area of skills makes fascinating reading. Porter states that 'In terms of general labour force skills, the UK still falls behind competing economies . . . [and] . . . UK companies report significant skill shortages that are consistent with these deficits.'

Porter turns his attention to the managerial workforce and, although he praises much of what he saw, he makes two telling points:

1 . . . UK companies adopt modern management techniques . . . later and less often than their competitors . . . [and] . . . they seem to achieve lower returns from implementing them.
2 Problems with management skills in the UK seem likely to be concentrated at the lower and middle management level, reflecting the overall skill deficit in the UK labour force.

It is only natural to respond to these findings by trying to 'rubbish the data'. We may well be tempted to say 'It's not like that in our healthcare organisation'. It may not be like that in your organisation, and you are to be congratulated if it is not, but if you remember the findings of the ORC opinion survey then it appears that Porter is right about all too many organisations.

This is one of the main reasons why I salute the Chartered Institute of Personnel and Development (CIPD) for the stance it is taking on the development of the notion of human capital. There are other reasons, too.

Towards intellectual capital

People Management has reported extensively on the former Department of Trade and Industry (DTI) consultation paper *Accounting for People*[13] and the task force it has established on human capital management. Its consultation paper was right to say that:

> it has become commonplace for business leaders to observe that 'our people are our greatest asset'. The skills and commitment of an organisation's people play a central role in delivering many of the factors most frequently identified as critical to continuing survival and success. But people are not passive 'assets', to be managed like any other asset. The performance of an organisation depends upon the motivation and commitment of its people as well as upon their knowledge and skills . . .
>
> Yet relatively few employers make a systematic attempt to assess their human capital (the relevant knowledge, skills, experience and learning capacity of the people available to the organisation), to appraise how well the organisation uses this resource through its HCM practices, or to examine changes over time.

However, the notion of human capital is merely one part of a much wider concept, and that is the idea of intellectual capital. Intellectual capital, and sometimes people use the phrase *knowledge management* to mean the same thing, is difficult to define but basically refers to human capital, the intelligence and data held within the organisation, and the various networks that an organisation can utilise. Michael Skapinker[14] summed it up nicely in the CIPD guide to knowledge management by defining it as: 'the ideas and experience of employees, customers and suppliers to improve the organisation's performance'.

Consider this extract taken from Thomas Stewart's *Intellectual Capital*:

> No executive would leave his cash or factory space idle, yet if CEOs are asked how much of the knowledge in their companies is used, they typically say 'About 20 per cent.' That is the observation of Betty Zucker, who studies knowledge management at the Gottlieb Duttweiler Foundation, a Swiss think tank. Says Zucker: 'Imagine the implications for a company if it could get that number up to just 30%.'[15]

And finally

Those of you who know something about the introduction of mass production into US manufacturing will be familiar with the story of Henry Ford. As he developed the introduction of production lines, with their serried ranks of assembly workers, it is claimed he once asked 'Why is it that whenever I ask for a pair of hands, a brain comes attached?'

Thankfully, we have advanced substantially since those days, and we realise the value to an organisation of its most important resource. But how far have we advanced? What if the survey figure of 50–60% is correct? Perhaps it is inaccurate, and maybe it should be 60% or even 70%. The truth is that none of us know. Whatever the true figure – 50%, 60% or 70% – there is still substantial scope for improvement.

How far have we advanced? Listen to these words of Andrew Carnegie:

> The only irreplaceable capital an organisation possesses is the knowledge and ability

of its people. The productivity of that capital depends on how effectively people share their competence with those who can use it.[16]

Three highly respected US academics have developed the notion of the *HR Scorecard*,[17] and their work emphasises the importance of understanding the fundamental point that the HR function does affect the 'bottom-line' performance of an organisation. Their work also provides HR practitioners with even more ammunition to show their organisations that HR work actually makes a positive and valuable contribution to the services that are being provided. The first quotation is profound:

> To paraphrase CK Prahalad and Gary Hamel, HR professionals are now in a position to become numerator managers (contributing to top-fine growth) rather than denominator managers (cutting costs and reducing overheads).

I believe that grasping the significance of this quotation will have a profound effect on the HR practitioner. For too long the world of HR management, or perhaps more accurately the world of personnel has been associated with productivity through a reduction in labour costs, and with cutting of numbers through efficiency measures – all *denominator* issues. Now there is a golden opportunity for the HR professional to realign and become associated with the development of the talent, the human capital within the organisation – the *numerator* issues. Some will protest at this assertion and remind me that for many years personnel professionals have been 'beavering away' at training and development issues, doing the very thing I am putting forward. If that is the assertion then it misses my point. Perhaps there have been enlightened individuals, though the status of training and development has hardly been influential, yet through the advent of the concept of intellectual capital there is an opportunity to secure a pivotal place for the HR function within the organisation. This is a different era – this is a new opportunity, and it is not the same as a reinvigorated training and development department.

This idea of aligning the HR function to developments in intellectual capital should be considered in tandem with writings on what have been called the 'soft' and 'hard' models of HR management. Truss[18] sets out these ideas, based to an extent on the writings of Guest, Storey and Legge, and shows that 'soft' models of HR management place the emphasis on the human part of the phrase, and as such are connected to the human relations school and the development of individual talents. 'Hard' models of HR management stress the management of the resource in a calculating and somewhat mechanistic manner. The fact that the term *HR management* can include such diagrammatically opposed approaches is surely one of its charms. As Truss comments, 'the soft perspective implies that individuals are viewed as a resource worthy of training and development, whereas the hard perspective implies that individuals are a cost to be minimised'.

The HR Scorecard authors argue:

The bottom line is this: if current accounting methods can't give HR professionals the measurement tools they need, then they will have to develop their own ways of demonstrating their contribution to firm performance. The first step is to discard the accounting mentality that says that HR is primarily a cost centre in which cost minimisation is the principal objective and measure of success. At the same time, HR managers must grasp the rare opportunity afforded them by this transitional period. Investors have made it clear that they value intangible assets. It's up to HR to develop a new measurement system that creates real value for the firm and secures human resources' legitimate place as a strategic partner.[19]

Are you getting the picture? The evidence to substantiate the key position of HR management is becoming overwhelming. Listen to the US academics: 'HR's emerging strategic potential hinges on the increasingly central role of intangible assets and intellectual capital in today's economy.' Then there are the UK academics Scarbrough and Elias:

> The economic conditions created by globalisation and the advent of new technologies have combined to make human capital and other intangible assets the major drivers of economic competitiveness. The increasingly critical role of these factors, however, has not been matched by advances in management and accounting practices.[20]

Becker and colleagues have a rightly deserved excellent reputation for their work, the idea of taking the highly regarded Scorecard[21] approach and applying it to the HR function is inspirational, and they make a number of valuable points that many will find a boon to their HR work. Although I found that their application appeared to become a little contrived at times, their book is worth investigating and might prove to be the answer for many an HR director who is struggling to demonstrate the added value of the department's contribution.

Jeffrey Pfeffer's[22] contribution to HR literature is highly commendable. He argues, in a chapter entitled 'The Business Case for Managing People Right', that his evidence shows 'substantial gains, of the order of 40 per cent or so, in most of the studies reviewed, can be obtained by implementing high-performance management practices'. This is some claim and, as if anticipating the incredulity of his readers, he adds '. . . these tremendous gains come about because high-commitment management approaches provide a number of important sources for enhanced organisational performance'. He identifies these high-commitment approaches as being concerned with systems of control, skills and competence, and greater responsibility being given to people (this is a very brief abbreviation on my part), and he elaborates on his evidence-based belief in a chapter entitled 'Seven Practices of Successful Organisations'.

In this chapter Pfeffer contends that the seven dimensions that seem to characterise most if not all of the systems that produce profits through people include employment security; self-managed teams and decentralisation of decision making; reduced status distinctions and barriers, and extensive sharing of financial and performance information.

Although I share his enthusiasm for each of these points, and believe that they can make a substantial difference to an organisation, I find myself siding with the CIPD's rather tactful comment that '. . . despite Pfeffer's assertions, there appears to be no single "one-size-fits-all" template that will work in every context'.[23]

The evidence is abundant, the arguments are persuasive and the case can be made – HR management has a substantial contribution to make to the 'bottom line'.

4 Understanding the importance of HR strategy

One of my pet hates is a writing style in which an article begins with a definition taken from a dictionary. The article usually starts with something along the lines 'As the *Oxford English Dictionary* (*OED*) tells us, the word "nerd" means . . .', and goes on to explain some fact that would have been far more interesting if a more imaginative style of writing had been employed.

I never thought that I would resort to this tactic, but when it comes to the word *strategy* I can think of no more fitting place to start. I need to define what I mean by the word *strategy*. It is one of those words that means all kinds of things to all kinds of people, yet it is used more often than not to imply important and high-level work, leaving the person hearing the word in a state of diffidence – unable to ask the speaker what exactly they meant by the word and in what context they were using it. To do so would place the questioner at an immediate disadvantage. Even if the user of the word did not say so, they would consider it a sad fact that in this day and age someone did not know the meaning of the word 'strategy'.

It is surprising to observe the number of people who have little or no grasp of strategy at all – they are the people who are happiest when they are 'doing things' (to use their phrase) or engaged in operational activity. This phenomenon can be seen in many meetings, often at senior levels, and it is alarming to observe the rapidity with which people move to a discussion of the minute details of operational matters and away from the big strategic picture.

My trusty *Chambers Dictionary* explains the word *strategy* as 'generalship, or the art of conducting a campaign and manoeuvring an army; artifice or finesse generally'. I know the word is sometimes used differently in management contexts – I have read enough of Professor Michael Porter to appreciate that point – but I am quite happy with my Chambers definition. As long as the military reference is converted into something that fits an organisation, the definition is perfectly adequate. For my use of the word, *strategy* concerns the big picture. It is about *conducting a campaign* within the organisation and *manoeuvring* its people, for the good of the organisation and in their interests, and doing so in an honourable manner and with some *finesse*, although there are times when it has to be done with a degree of *artifice*.

The best description of strategy in the HR context comes from the work of Sisson and Storey[24] who, in a pragmatic and down-to-earth way, show that 'typically, a more strategic approach [to HR management] is seen as embracing [some of] the following: regarding people as a strategic resource for achieving competitive advantage, a coherent approach to employment policies and practices, and proactive rather than reactive management.'

Storey takes this notion a step further in his introduction to another text,[25] and demonstrates that 'HRM . . . to some extent . . . can be regarded also as an attempted articulation of an alternative to the Fordist-IR model of labour management which aimed to secure compliance through temporary truces based on negotiated settlements.' He identifies 12 key elements of the 'new' alternative approach under the sub-headings of beliefs and assumptions, strategic qualities, the critical role of managers, and key levers.

So how do HR professionals engage in strategy? The starting point has to be the classic Harvard approach set out in *Managing Human Assets*.[26] I know this is a dated text, but I would argue that it has stood the test of time, and the fact that it is reproduced in a range of HR books suggests that most people find it a helpful starting point. As I help clients to write HR strategies for their organisations, it is the Harvard diagram and text that they as practitioners find the most useful starting point and although they are hardly likely to place the diagram in their strategies, the thinking provoked by it is clearly seen. The way in which it interweaves stakeholder interests, situational factors and the development of HR management policy choices, HR outcomes and long-term consequences is seen as being inspirational and extremely helpful. Beer's words resonate with practitioner experience, and they concur with his view that the traditional problems of personnel can be best solved:

> . . . when general managers develop a viewpoint of how they wish to see employees involved in and developed by the enterprise, and of what HRM policies and practices might achieve these goals. Without either a central philosophy or a strategic view – which can be provided only by general managers – HRM is likely to remain a set of independent activities, each guided by its own practice tradition.[27]

The approach of Beer and colleagues helps HR professionals to think about the 'big picture', the wider context in which the HR function will operate, and the approach's four Cs (*commitment, competence, cost-effectiveness* and *congruence*) remain as relevant today as when they were first identified.

The work may be dated, and some of their principles appear to be more concerned with the *denominator* approach to HR management rather than the *numerator* approach advocated earlier, but they are a part of the classic inheritance that the HR function possesses, and should form the basis of most engagements assessing the impact of HR strategy. I agree with Boxall's view that (some of) the advantages of this model are that it incorporates recognition of a range of stakeholder interests, it widens the context of HR management to include 'employee influence' and it acknowledges a broad range of contextual influences on management's choice of strategy.[28]

HR managers who are faced with a challenge to 'be strategic' could do far worse than place the six questions posed by Ulrich[29] on their desks when asked to ensure that their work is properly linked to the organisational outcomes. His analytical questions challenge the HR practitioner to examine strategy critically, and they refer to the organisation's shared mind-set, competence, consequence (appropriate rewards and measures), governance, capacity for change and leadership.

5 Check out the quality and roles of your HR professionals

My third initial proposition was that *the key determinant of effectiveness and relevance in the HR function is the quality of its own professional staff*. A lifetime of experience has taught me that this is an essential factor. When you think about this for a few moments it becomes a self-evident truth. If the HR department is staffed by bright, motivated people who know what they are doing and understand the needs of the organisation, it is far less likely that anyone is going to question the worth of the department to the organisation. Conversely, if the HR department is staffed by deadbeats whom no one else rates highly, and the work of HR staff seems to be tangential to the work of the organisation, then it is likely that many questions are going to be asked about the merits of that particular department.

The most eloquent exposition of this point comes again from the pen of Dave Ulrich.[30] He puts forward the view that HR management can help to deliver organisational excellence in four ways, which can be conveniently summarised as becoming a partner with senior and line managers in strategy execution, delivering administrative efficiency, becoming a champion for employees, and becoming an agent of continuous transformation. This is a challenging and highly commendable agenda for HR management, and it is quite clear that this agenda can only be delivered by competent people who are dedicated to the performance of the organisation, and who are respected by their peers and bosses. Ulrich goes further and, drawing on research, he puts forward the view that as HR management comes increasingly to be viewed as a profession, there is a need for HR professionals who are able to, among other things, know the organisation, master HR practices, manage change processes and demonstrate personal credibility.

The point has been made. This can only be achieved by equipping the HR department with the brightest and the best.

6 Discover the utility of the psychological contract

Each year one of the Sunday broadsheet newspapers conducts a survey to discover the employer of the year. It has developed a set of criteria for this prestigious honour, and by surveying the employees of various organisations it decides which organisation should receive the award. One of the most impressive features of the award is that it is the employees of the organisation who vote on the merits of the employer. Although the overall assessment process may resemble a popularity competition more than a serious statistical survey, no one can gainsay the fact that large numbers of employees consider their employer to be the best in the UK. Each year I look at the results and am surprised by the fact that organisations which are not known for their high wages (e.g. a particular supermarket chain) can nonetheless perform exceptionally well in the survey, and some organisations whose wages are high can do poorly. It substantiates the age-old point that it is not only pay that determines an employee's contentment with an organisation and that it is possible to pay low wages – not that I am advocating this – and still have a contented workforce.

This is one of the major reasons why the idea of the psychological contract is so important. The psychological contract can be best defined as:

> the perceptions of both parties to the employment relationship, organisation and individual, of the reciprocal promises and obligations implied in that relationship. Put more simply, both workers and their employers believe that they have certain basic obligations to the other, and that these should be reciprocated in some way.[31]

It is possible for an HR professional to examine a model of the psychological contract, a model based on academic theory and practical experience, and to consider:

➤ a set of background organisational and individual factors
➤ a set of policy influences and work experiences
➤ a system that attempts to measure the state of the psychological contract
➤ a set of attitudinal and behavioural outcomes.

The instrument does not claim to be a precise mathematical tool, but it does provide the HR director with a methodology whereby the health of the organisation, as judged by the relationships of worker and employer, can be assessed. There are well-known organisations that have succeeded in taking their needs and the needs of their employees and producing a symmetrical or congruent approach to the management of human resources with the result that both parties – the organisation and the employees – are extremely content, the modern-day equivalent of expressing the notion of 'peace and efficiency', well known to students of industrial relations in the 1960s and 1970s. Other organisations, experiencing an almost identical environment and offering their employees identical terms and conditions of employment, seem to be incapable of achieving the ideal of a psychological contract that appears to be in balance, an environment in which all agree that the organisation is a good place to work. One organisation can do it and the other cannot. The role of the HR function in these circumstances is clear, and each HR professional has a responsibility to ensure that they can achieve suitable conditions for the sake of the employees and the organisation.

7 Set out to achieve best fit rather than best practice

Anyone who has been associated with the benchmarking and re-engineering revolutions is likely to have trawled around their own and other countries looking for examples of best practice. The perennial questions were 'Why can they make it cheaper than us?' or 'Why can they turn around a product or service 30% faster than us?' or Why are they, with the same equipment and staffing as us, 15% more productive than we are?' These are important questions, especially in a global-market environment, and the answers have had an impact on improving the economic prosperity of organisations and countries.

However, there was a drawback. Some organisations went in search of the best-performing organisations in the world, in search of the best management practices, and brought them back to their organisation without any recognition of the cultural differences between different nations and organisations, and without any sense of whether they would have to adapt what they had witnessed elsewhere. I can well remember one senior executive who returned to his organisation following a visit to the USA. With a cigar in his mouth he started his meeting by declaring, in mid-Atlantic drawl, 'What you guys need to do is . . .' His team nearly fell about laughing, but then thought better of such open opposition to his new-found ideas. Another executive I knew well spent four weeks in Japan studying their approach to quality management, and experienced a personal conversion. He went there sceptical about the claims being made, but returned as a disciple of their approach to management, especially quality management. What he had seen influenced him immensely, and what he said about the need to change practice in his organisation was absolutely right, but he failed to appreciate fully the need to make his message culturally sensitive. He was listened to politely, as you would expect in relation to someone of his seniority, but within a relatively short time he became sidelined within the organisation. His continuous references to Japan grated on the other managers and, over time, even irritated his boss who had sent him there in the first place. There is a danger of finding best practice and then trying to mimic it within another context without paying attention to the cultural niceties. Fortunately, HR academics and practitioners appear to be aware of these dangers. The following three examples demonstrate the lessons learned, and should be taken to heart by HR professionals everywhere. The first example comes from the work of Armstrong and Baron:

> . . . it is accepted by most commentators that 'best fit' is more important than 'best practice'. There can be no universal prescriptions for HRM policies and practices. It all depends. This is not to say that 'good practice' or 'leading-edge practice' – i.e. practice that does well in one successful environment – should be ignored. Benchmarking has its uses as a means of identifying areas for innovation or development that are practised to good effect elsewhere by leading companies. But having learned about what works and, ideally, what does not work in comparable organisations, it is up to the firm to decide what may be relevant in general terms and what lessons can be learned that can be adapted to fit its own particular strategic and operational requirements.[32]

The second quote is taken from the seminal CIPD report, *Understanding the People and Performance Link*:

> Organisations seeking to optimise the contribution that people management can make must develop policies and practices that meet the needs of individuals and create 'a great place to work'. However, this does not just mean copying 'best practice'. Organisations must create and transmit values and culture which are unique to themselves, which bind the organisation together, and which can be measured and managed.[33]

The final quote is taken from an extensive report on the change agenda in the public sector and the importance of engaging, empowering and energising people.[34] The researchers examined six public-sector organisations and drew out important HR management practices from which all organisations can benefit, but in their final section, entitled 'No two journeys are the same', they add:

> The research has made it very clear that every change process involves a unique journey that reflects the starting point, the goals, the people, culture, history and context of each organisation. Therefore other organisations that are seeking to learn from this journey will only ever have a partial, retrospective picture of what was done, what was learned and what was ultimately achieved.

The message could hardly be clearer. HR practitioners need to discover best practice from other organisations, and from academics or consultants, and it is essential that they adapt these best practices to fit the needs of their organisation. Only then are they ensuring that HR practice is tailored to the needs of the organisation and the other strategies by which the organisation is steered.

Key actions

1 You need to identify the principles and values that underpin your view of HR management, and develop policies and actions that make a real difference to your people and your healthcare organisation.

2 As a believer in effective HR management do not be slow to make your views known. HR management has much to offer, and by showing both the 'hard' and the 'soft' side, the 'numerator' and the 'denominator' approach, you will enable your colleagues to understand the value of effective HR management.

3 Become a real HR expert, be concerned about the way in which staff are led, and demonstrate how much you add to the quality of the healthcare services that are being provided.

REFERENCES

1 West MA, Borrill C, Dawson J, *et al.* (2002) The link between the management of employees and patient mortality in acute hospitals. *International Journal of Human Resource Management.* 13(8): 1299–310.

2 Ibid.

3 Ibid.

4 Legge K (1995) *Human Resource Management. Rhetoric and realities.* Palgrave, Basingstoke.

5 Ritzer G and Trice HM (1969) *An Occupation in Conflict.* Cornell University Press, New York.

6 Storey J (1992) *Developments in the Management of Human Resources.* Blackwell, Oxford.

7 Guest D, Michie J, Sheehan M, *et al.* (2000) *Effective People Management.* Research Report. Chartered Institute of Personnel and Development, London.

8 Purcell J, Kinnie N, Hutchinson S, *et al.* (2003) *Understanding the People and*

Performance Link: unlocking the black box. Research Report. Chartered Institute of Personnel and Development, London.

9 Organisation for Economic Co-operation and Development (OECD) (1996) *Measuring What People Know: human capital accounting for the knowledge economy.* OECD, Paris.

10 Bontis N (1998) Intellectual capital: an exploratory study. *Manag Decision.* 36(2): 63–76.

11 Scarbrough H and Elias J (2002) *Evaluating Human Capital.* Research Report. Chartered Institute of Personnel and Development, London.

12 Ibid.

13 *Accounting for People*; Department of Trade and Industry website. www.dti.org

14 Skapinker M (2002) *Knowledge Management.* Research Report. Chartered Institute of Personnel and Development, London.

15 Stewart TA (1998) *Intellectual Capital.* Nicholas Brealey, London.

16 Ibid.

17 Becker BE, Huselid MA and Ulrich D (2001) *The HR Scorecard.* Harvard Business School Press, Boston, MA.

18 Truss C (1999) Soft and hard models of human resource management. In: L Gratton, VH Hailey, P Stiles and C Truss (eds) *Strategic Human Resource Management.* Oxford University Press, Oxford.

19 Becker BE, Huselid MA and Ulrich D (2001) *The HR Scorecard.* Harvard Business School Press, Boston, MA.

20 Scarbrough H and Elias J (2002) *Evaluating Human Capital.* Research Report. Chartered Institute of Personnel and Development, London.

21 Becker BE, Huselid MA and Ulrich D (2001) *The HR Scorecard.* Harvard Business School Press, Boston, MA.

22 Pfeffer J (1998) *The Human Equation.* Harvard Business School Press, Boston, MA.

23 Caulkin S (2001) *Performance Through People.* Research Report. Chartered Institute of Personnel and Development, London.

24 Sisson K and Storey J (2000) *The Realities of Human Resource Management.* Open University Press, Buckingham.

25 Storey J (ed.) (2001) *Human Resource Management: a critical text.* Thomson, London.

26 Beer M, Spector B, Lawrence P, *et al.* (1984) *Managing Human Assets.* Harvard Business School Press, Boston, MA.

27 Ibid.

28 Boxall PF (1992) Strategic HRM: a beginning, a new theoretical direction. *Human Resource Manag J.* 6(3): 59–75.

29 Ulrich D (1998) *A New Mandate for Human Resources.* (Harvard Business Review). Harvard Business School Press, Boston, MA.

30 Ulrich D (1999) *Delivering Results: a new mandate for human resource professionals.* Harvard Business School Press, Boston, MA.

31 Guest DE and Conway N (2002) *Pressure at Work and the Psychological Contract.* Research Report. Chartered Institute of Personnel and Development, London.

32 Armstrong M and Baron A (2002) *Strategic HRM.* Chartered Institute of Personnel and Development, London.

33 Purcell J, Kinnie N, Hutchinson S, *et al.* (2003) *Understanding the People and Performance Link: unlocking the black box.* Research Report. Chartered Institute of Personnel and Development, London.

34 Vere D and Beaton L (2003) *Delivering Public Services: the change agenda*. Research Report. Chartered Institute of Personnel and Development, London.

FURTHER READING

Bach S and Sisson K (eds) (2000) *Personnel Management. A comprehensive guide to theory and practice*. Blackwell Business, Oxford.

Attitudes

CHAPTER 6

Being patient focused

It may appear unusual, in a book written primarily for those engaged in health-care, to write a chapter encouraging you to be patient focused in all actions. The reason for writing such a chapter is based on my experiences as a patient and the positive reaction I have received from various clinicians, healthcare academics, managers and policy makers, from many countries, when I have shared my experiences with them. Although difficult to believe, it is possible to be so engrossed in the actual delivery of healthcare, with all its challenges and pressures, that the particular needs of the individual patient can be missed or not seen as having great importance. This is not intentional myopia on the part of clinicians and managers but rather a case of sometimes not being able to see the wood for the trees.

In this chapter I set out a number of challenges for general and clinical management, in response to what I term the 'curse of unplanned and unhelpful variation'. The chapter ends by asking why colleagues I have encountered, from various professions and countries, recognise the validity of these challenges and yet have few solutions when it comes to removing the 'curse'.

BEDS AND BATHS

When I worked in the health service one of my colleagues, who had started her career as a trainee hotel manager, used to tell amusing tales about her days in the hotel trade. One of those anecdotes remains fresh in my memory and is relevant to my experience as patient.

One of her numerous responsibilities was to check that the chambermaids and cleaners had left each room in a pristine condition: each bed had to be made and every room cleaned against a strict, laid-down standard. After all, this was a four-star hotel with aspirations of five-star status. The hotel's general manager told her there was only one way to inspect that standards were being maintained in the bedrooms: you had to lie down on the bed, and in the bath, to have the same view as the guests and to be able to check if there were any embarrassing stains, cobwebs, or unclean spots anywhere in the room. And she went off to lie down in 50 or 60 baths and beds, week after week. You will see the relevance of this anecdote immediately.

Between 1996 and 2006 I was an in-patient in six hospitals and a regular outpatient in two others. I might have been a health service employee for 20 years, but it was only when I spent time in hospital beds and baths that I was able to gain valuable insight that only patients can obtain. I have seen it all: the good, the bad and the just about acceptable and this may be the account of a former health service manager, and a current academic, but above all it is the account of a patient – a patient who can look at the health service through a relevant diagnostic lens.

It is the account of a patient who is an ardent supporter of the health service. What is written is fair and balanced: the dedication and accomplishments of clinicians and other staff are acknowledged – they did, after all, twice save my life and I owe them a debt I shall never be able to repay and the depth and extent of my gratitude is hard to communicate on paper.

THE CURSE OF VARIATION

Ask anyone responsible for providing quality services and they will explain that the greatest obstacle to the provision of consistent first-rate services is the curse of unacceptable and unplanned variation: sometimes the service is excellent, sometimes adequate; sometimes staff perform superbly, at other times they are quite ordinary, or even inadequate. For some reason, one part of the organisation can deliver excellence in everything it does; yet other parts cannot muster the necessary level of consistency to meet the needs of its clients. In all organisations, managers realise that unacceptable variation – the antithesis of 'conformance to standard', rather than acceptable variation that adds spice to life – has to be tackled.

As a patient, I was surprised by the unacceptable and unplanned variations existing between hospitals, within the same hospital, occasionally between and within the same professions, and sometimes on the same ward. To illustrate this variability of service here are a number of questions based on my experience.

➤ Why is it that some hospitals have highly efficient administrative services in terms, for example, of the letters sent to the patient, and others are consistently poor?

➤ Why are some receptionists pleasant and helpful and others miserable and grudging?

➤ Why don't equally skilled people undertake tests?

➤ Why don't all staff realise how vulnerable patients feel, how worried they are, and how much they need hospital staff to be supportive?

➤ Why do some doctors seem to believe that the less a patient is told, the better?

➤ Why are some nurses distant, rather than friendly, and only do something to make the patient comfortable when asked to do it?

➤ Why can one hospital provide decent, edible food, ordered a few hours before being served, yet another hospital can only offer poor food, ordered by another patient who occupied the bed two days previously?

➤ Why are some bathroom facilities clean and reasonable and other facilities deplorable?

➤ And, above all, why is it that in a health service where surgeons and others perform consistently at world-class standards, other dimensions of the service are merely good-to-adequate or, worse still, mediocre-to-poor?

I have not even mentioned variations in clinical practice but the examples are sufficient to make my point. This variation is widespread, needs addressing and eradication, and is one of the greatest patient experience challenges facing healthcare managers. If unplanned and unacceptable variation were eradicated, wherever possible, it would lead to substantial improvement in the quality of health services and benefit the patient significantly. Most improvements would be cost neutral, as most of what I observed and recommend involves sound management practice, the type of sound practice that good hospitals, or even good wards within moderate hospitals, already practise. I have categorised these observations under the headings of six key issues.

KEY ISSUE #1: THE RECORDING OF INFORMATION

We live in the information age. If I *Google*™ my medical condition, 900 000 references appear in 0.18 seconds; if I buy something over the telephone my postcode and Visa card allows the supplier to access an immense amount of information; and when I buy books from Amazon, typing my password onto an electronic order form initiates their invoicing and mailing systems.

Information in the health service is a source of amazement to the patient. Hospitals are not made up of technophobes – the array of computerised clinical equipment bears testimony to that – it is just that so many of the administrative systems and procedures are archaic. There are reams of papers, bulging files, and a plethora of handwritten and sometimes indecipherable comments. All of this would be fine if the systems were highly efficient – the patient would be willing to smile approvingly at those good old ways of doing things – but the patient's concern is that the systems lack the robustness and effectiveness experienced in other areas of life and necessary in the best interests of the patient.

These problems are acknowledged in various official documents, identifying issues for professionals and patients. For professionals: delays in getting results because they are paper based; poor access to evidence in the workplace; time-consuming recording by hand in patient notes; frustration at the unavailability of notes produced by others; and errors caused by poor access to timely information. For patients: wasted journeys because records are mislaid; frustration as the same information is requested again and again; inconvenience and discomfort through repeat tests when results are lost; anxiety through lack of continuity and clear explanation; and incorrect treatment due to mis-identification or mis-diagnosis.

The patient's experience would be improved substantially if there were a record of their medical history and treatment available to the clinicians once the patient has been identified. Without such a system, the patient is relied upon to describe not only current symptoms – which seems perfectly reasonable and without alternative – but also the history of treatment in other hospitals. This description of previous treatment has to be given repeatedly to various clinicians, as they appear unable to share the first description. It is reasonable to be asked as many diagnostic questions as are necessary but what is unreasonable is to be required to repeat the same facts over and over again. What is more, to repeat one's story at a time when the patient may be in severe pain, possibly confused and definitely worried about the future is not a pleasant experience. There is also the worrying feeling that the efficacy of one's care might depend, somehow, on how well one is able to draw on powers of memory and articulation at a time of great need and stress.

Then there is the issue of sharing planned diagnostic information. Most patients are willing to travel for treatment by the most appropriate clinician. However, this willingness to travel is not always extended to the matter of routine and planned diagnostic tests. Why is it ever necessary to undertake a six- or eight-hour round trip to be X-rayed, CT scanned, MRI-ed, or to have blood taken? Why cannot those tests be undertaken in the patient's local hospital and the 'raw' results (even if not the definitive interpretation of those results) be sent electronically to the clinicians in the hospital some distance away? Would this not be the most economical alternative and certainly the most environmentally friendly procedure at a time when people are concerned about carbon footprints? There might be administrative hurdles to overcome and there may be occasions when the tests need to be undertaken in the same hospital as the planned treatment for clinical reasons, but in all other circumstances the economic and patient-friendly route should come first.

IT technophiles will claim the answer lies in some sophisticated multi-billion pound computer system, and well it might, but I am aware of the problems encountered by public bodies (and others) when they embark upon expensive computer solutions. My observation calls for a far less sophisticated solution which has more to do with the management of information, probably with the support of local PCs, laptops and hand-held computers, rather than with elaborate, expensive and potentially calamitous universal information systems.

KEY ISSUE #2: SERVICES THAT ARE CONNECTED ONE TO ANOTHER

It is a first-class experience when the various components of the hospital system are co-ordinated, allowing the patient to move seamlessly from one department to another. There will be occasional delays, to allow for emergencies or schedules falling behind time, but generally the patient feels expected in every department and the members of the department know what test or treatment to give the patient. It's a case of the 'left hand' of the system knowing what the 'right hand' is doing and the patient being the benefactor of that co-ordination.

Whilst most hospitals would gain a general pass mark for the connectivity of their services, it is all too easy to falsely assume that every single service in the hospital works with precision. That is clearly not the case. Although hospital professionals and services operate efficiently within their particular domain, within their sphere of activity (such as physiotherapy, radiology, surgery, specialist nursing, or whatever), they do not always ensure that the individual services are fully connected. In other words, far too many services are disconnected and the patient experiences the parts not properly joined together.

Some examples illustrate this point.

➤ A patient turns up for a session of physiotherapy and the physiotherapist is not sure what they are expected to do with the patient as they cannot understand the doctor's handwriting.

➤ Some catering teams realise the therapeutic value of a good cup of tea and nourishing food, coupled with a cheerful disposition and appropriate banter, and some teams are the complete opposite: they make little contact with the patient, even manage to place the therapeutic cup of tea just out of reach and possess little sense of the importance of their role.

➤ In some hospitals a patient is given a supply of medication within a short time of the doctor saying they can go home. In other hospitals the medication can take up to seven hours to arrive.

➤ One day-patient experience stands out. The procedure was undertaken in modern facilities, the nursing care was excellent, I cannot praise the doctors highly enough for their skill and the way they spoke to me throughout the whole procedure. It was an excellent experience, a credit to the hospital and its staff. And yet, I was asked to change into a surgical gown in the nearby gentleman's toilet – a room that was small and smelly, and near the reception desk so somewhat public.

➤ How was it possible for an orthopaedic surgeon to perform surgery on me – only for the regional specialists (located in another hospital in the same organisation) and a national orthopaedic specialist to question the legitimacy of the procedure?

➤ My worst experience took place in a highly regarded hospital, with top-class clinicians and management. I needed a test urgently and was taken to the diagnostic facilities in my bed by two porters. When I arrived I was told there was a delay of approximately 40 minutes. The porters parked my bed in the corridor, outside the suite, and left as they had another patient to move. I was left on my own and in a corridor that was, in effect, a public thoroughfare: many outpatients and visitors made their way down that corridor. I had been given pain killers on the ward and after a short while fell asleep and woke up, about 90 minutes later, still unattended, to find my wife sitting at the foot of the bed. She'd been there for about 40 minutes, which meant I had been on my own for 40 or 50 minutes. Eventually, the nurse and consultant greeted me and treated me wonderfully. This is the perfect example of the lack of connectivity that often takes place. The doctor and nurses on the ward were doing their job expertly when they sent me on my way; the porters did an excellent job in wheeling me down and avoiding the bumps to ease my pain; the diagnostic staff could not have given me better care. And yet there was a yawning gap in the overall system that allowed me to lie in a bed, in a public corridor, in pain and on my own for over an hour (if my wife hadn't turned up when she did). To be charitable, it is possible that someone was keeping an eye on me, but I was not aware of it and neither was my wife.

Anyone who has witnessed clinical staff working in their single or multi-professional teams cannot fail to be impressed. In order for effective surgery to take place the most complex team arrangements have to function with an attention to intricate detail. Throughout the hospital systems, teams of professionals work to the highest standards, but problems arise in the 'white space' between these teams and there are times when the patient falls between the equivalent of two or three stools.

Ensuring that the whole system works effectively is a key senior management task. If the hospital has an organisation chart, or a variety of flow diagrams on which every box is square and every circle perfectly round and every arrow straight and each part of the organisation joined to some other part, then the management should be alarmed: they should throw away the charts and diagrams and walk around the hospital and talk to the patients. The charts and diagrams are probably misleading – everything is certainly not symmetrical and smooth from the perspective of the patient. Managers should go and discover how the 'white spaces' on the charts might contain a variety of practices unknown to senior management, or how the regular design of systems is actually incongruent with what takes place on a daily basis.

KEY ISSUE #3: THE RELATIONSHIP BETWEEN THE PATIENT AND THE CLINICIAN

The principle of unacceptable variation can be present in the relationship between the patient and the clinician. Take the example of nursing. Typically, nurses are expert, hard working and more than willing to take time to answer questions to increase the patient's knowledge or to allay fears. There is also a kaleidoscope of different *cultures, personalities, organisations* and even *practices*. This is hardly surprising given their number, and as the patient is in their presence *24/7*, as they say.

In terms of *practice* I think of nurses who were highly professional, operating at what seemed like the cutting-edge of technology and clinical practice, who played a major role in ensuring my recovery; and nurses who appeared solely to perform administrative tasks on behalf of doctors. I am also aware that a full range of nursing activities can be enormously helpful to the patient: one nurse, who had provided me with 'high-tech' care, made me drinking chocolate and toast at 3.30 in the morning, a meal that signalled I had just turned the corner in my recovery.

It is inevitable and welcome that the *personalities* of nurses should differ. Every personality type imaginable can be found and – although this is inevitable – there are occasions when a patient's inability to 'read' the best way to ask a nurse for something can be disadvantageous. This is one of the reasons that patients in some hospitals wait, with eager anticipation, to see which group of nurses will be taking care of them for the next 8- or 12-hour shift. In blunt language, some nurses are easier to get on with than others and seem to take better care of you.

Diversity is an apt word to describe the individual *cultures* to be found on a ward, especially in the larger city hospitals. I overheard one sister tell a colleague from another ward that her six staff nurses for the night shift came from six different overseas countries. No doubt such diversity is to be welcomed, especially as it brings to the country some gifted and caring nurses (although there are concerns over the corresponding decrease in talent within their home countries), but some have a command of English that leaves much to be desired.

Then there are the different *organisations* and the unsurprising fact that these can differ quite markedly and that key individuals on the ward establish the tone of the place, the organisational culture. I have been fortunate in that the majority of nurses who have looked after me have been both professional and friendly, have provided excellent care and at the same time have been able to cheer up the patient. But the differences between hospitals are worth mentioning. Some manage to be professional and warm and friendly, whilst others can only manage the professional side of that equation and there can be significant difficulties in the nature of care received.

Understanding the mindset of the patient helps to set events in a proper context. Most patients feel vulnerable: they are, after all, in a strange environment, away from their families, potentially embarrassed by what they have to take part in (the commode!), possibly in pain and anxious about what the doctors are going to tell them on their next ward round. Patients, in such a state, need to be treated with kid gloves. My experience is that this is not always the case. I would not want to be called a 'customer'; that would be unnatural and the patient–clinician relationship should never be similar to that between an individual and a car salesman, but it would do no harm if some clinicians were taught to think of their patients as customers – in this way the common decencies of relationships could be improved.

KEY ISSUE #4: THE ON-GOING TRAINING AND DEVELOPMENT OF STAFF

The patient has three main requirements of the people charged with taking care of them.

1 A professional and practical competence

One assumes that the uniform worn by the person is an indication of their competence. It means they are professionally qualified; they have been accredited; they are subject to the diktats of a regulatory body; they are committed to keeping their knowledge and skills up-to-date, and they can apply their knowledge practically.

The patient does not believe that all staff in a professional group are, or need to be, equally qualified or even equally competent; but patients do believe there is a basic level of qualification and competence below which no person charged with looking after them is allowed to fall. It seems to be a reasonable assumption and a fundamental area of trust to expect those charged with caring for the patient to be competent.

If the patient trusts staff to be competent and aware of latest developments in their profession, then it behoves the individuals concerned to ensure they live up to the faith placed in them. A patient readily accepts that one nurse, or one doctor, may be more knowledgeable or more skilful or more experienced than another, but the patient should not tolerate a clinician who claims to be a professional and yet does little to maintain their level of knowledge and practice. The patient does not want to be looked after by a surgeon 10 years out of date, or a nurse who fails to keep up with latest practice, or a hospital manager who resembles an old-fashioned administrator.

2 A compassionate and caring nature

Any patient facing a test or procedure, even one they have gone through previously in the same hospital, is still nervous and wonders: Will the procedure go well? Will the results be okay? Is this the final test before I start living a more normal life?

I can think of one test I had, a test I'd had on half a dozen previous occasions in the same hospital, where the procedures bordered on the edge of being farcical. As the needle was inserted, blood from my arm squirted high into the air; and the equipment set up for the next stage of the test had been inserted incorrectly, and I was sprayed with a harmless liquid. A charming diagnostician, who had not mastered the procedures, caused this to happen; fortunately I was able to laugh it off but afterwards felt distressed by the experience. Again, the curse of variation: when someone who should have been supervised was left alone to administer a normally routine procedure. This example shows the need for professional and practical competence in addition to compassion and charm.

Being compassionate and caring also extends to the difference between a clinician reacting to a request for care and one taking a proactive role in making the patient comfortable and ensuring that their needs are met to the best of their ability. A patient understands quickly: some clinicians should only be asked for help when absolutely essential; others are more than happy to help with every reasonable need.

3 A personality allowing the patient to develop an appropriate relationship

Everyone understands that no two clinicians are identical; they have different backgrounds, interests and personalities. What one clinician considers a suitable approach may not suit others who are more or less introvert or extrovert. What is true of a clinician is also true of a patient: no two patients are identical and their needs, the ways they express themselves, or the ways they wish to be dealt with, should be taken into account. Some hospital wards are expert in the way they treat patients and other wards treat all patients as if they were exactly the same. Variation can occur on the same ward, between one clinician and another, where one takes into account the preferences of the patient and another fails to see the need for helpful discrimination. This, in turn, makes it difficult for the patient to know exactly how to deal with their relationship with a clinician and their preferred modes of functioning.

Naturally, the patient allows the individual caring for them to know many personal details and often the patient is at their most vulnerable. Most clinicians manage to create proper relationship but there are those who fail; they may not even see the need for such a relationship. There are times when hospital systems, such as shift rota patterns, militate against the development of such appropriate relationships and the patient has to form relationships with numerous different (in style, practice and temperament) individuals.

KEY ISSUE #5: THE SKILL OF COMMUNICATION

Despite the fact that there is nothing wrong with my hearing or reasoning, there have been occasions when I failed to understand the significance of an important point being made by a clinician – usually my wife had to interject. In normal circumstances I would have picked up the point immediately, been aware of the nuances and implications, but in hospital, experiencing the after-effects of medication and anaesthesia, coupled with fear and pain, there are times when an important piece of information is not understood. Therefore, clinicians who double-check that their message has been understood are an added bonus.

The following four examples of poor and good communication have been chosen carefully from dozens of such examples. They show that communication is not some God-given gift; they acknowledge that some people are better at it than others, and the examples of poor communication are based on issues that, significantly, are systemic within some hospitals. The examples also demonstrate two important principles: first, there are times when the wrong person in the organisation makes a communication; second, poor communication can take place because of an inefficient or unthinking individual.

Example 1 – As I was being wheeled out of one hospital, after a long stay in its wards, a nursing auxiliary said to my wife and me: *'It's so good to see you going home, especially after you came so close.'* 'So close', I thought to myself, *'whatever does she mean?'* I asked what she meant. *'Well, you know,'* she said *'so close, when you nearly didn't go home.'* This was news to me. No one else from the ward had said this, even though it had dawned on me as a distinct possibly, especially during the early part of my stay. But this was the first time that anyone from the ward had said it to me and it came as a surprise. But I let the matter drop and wished her well. I was delighted to be going home.

Example 2 – I turned up in outpatients for what I thought was an annual routine appointment with a consultant, expecting to be told that everything was fine and that he would see me again in 12 months' time. As I sat in a consultation room a friendly nursing assistant took my blood pressure and handed me a manual *'that I give to everyone about to have surgery'.* I have to confess that I was feeling a little tetchy that afternoon; it was warm, I was tired after a long drive through heavy traffic, and said: *'What do you mean "surgery"? I'm not having surgery'.* She disappeared and an experienced sister appeared and said something about handing out manuals being a routine procedure. Thirty minutes later I emerged from the hospital, in a daze, after the consultant had explained that I needed surgery. I apologised to the sister for my earlier tetchiness and left the hospital with my head spinning as I thought about what I had to face.

The third example concerns those occasions when oral communication is misunderstood, misinterpreted or downright wrong. An ambulance was taking me to the local accident and emergency department. The ambulance man was an engaging type, and may have been trained to talk to the patient to keep their minds off the pain they were feeling; the discussions ranged wide, including his liberal views on cannabis. He explained: *'GPs expect me to give you X* [some medication] *to ease the pain while in the ambulance, but I don't do that because if I did then when you get to the hospital the A&E staff won't be able to give you all of their pain relief stuff'.* When we arrived in A&E I was put on a trolley, wheeled in and greeted by the sister. The ambulance man briefed the sister and said: *'I've given Mr Prosser X to ease his pain'. 'Oh no you haven't'*, I shouted, and he responded: *'Oh no, I haven't given Mr Prosser anything'.* And with that turned and walked out; the sister muttered something under her breath.

The final example demonstrates the power of non-verbal communication. It came at a time when some people thought I might not be long for this world. I remember three consultants and two specialist registrars standing at the foot of my bed, with the curtains drawn and four of them looking glum. They shared some comments with one another, then spoke pleasantly but solemnly to me, and started to leave my cubicle. As the final one left – he was one of the registrars – he turned, gave me a large smile and thumbs up signal, and playfully punched my foot. I'll never forget that moment and the feeling that perhaps one doctor thought I might just pull through my current difficulties. Perhaps he did not, but his actions certainly boosted my confidence. That was a powerful example of positive and intimate non-verbal communication.

KEY ISSUE #6: THE INVISIBLE HAND OF SENIOR MANAGEMENT

The typical patient has no idea what hospital managers do. Such a lack of understanding may not bother hospital managers who see themselves as hidden assets, beavering away to ensure that a multitude of different components come together enabling those on the front line to deliver services. And, in many ways, such an attitude demonstrates the admirable qualities of the hospital management ethos.

Worryingly, it is not only patients who have little idea how senior managers spend their time – a large number of front-line staff do not know what senior managers do. Usually, they know what their immediate boss does but there is little understanding or recognition of the crucial role played by senior management in ensuring the smooth running of the hospital and the wider organisation. This is one of the reasons that some clinicians join conversations with patients eulogising the role of ward staff and criticising the role of senior management. Sometimes it is done innocently or naively; at other times there is a willingness to disparage senior management bordering on disloyalty.

Perhaps this is not surprising. Senior managers spend much of their time in little direct contact with ward-based activities; yet without senior management actions the ward activities would be impossible to undertake. Within the health system the role of senior management in strategy, financial management, human resources, dealing with government, and much else involved in running a healthcare establishment, is indispensable.

I believe healthcare managers to be hardworking, dedicated and caring. However, as a patient I believe senior managers should re-arrange their priorities to enable them to deal with issues of unacceptable variations in service delivery and to tackle these issues in a manner that shows clearly their contribution to front-line healthcare delivery. Senior managers should be more involved in ward-based matters, in those priorities for patients, and less involved in developing further policies and attending even more meetings.

Would it not make sense for senior managers to be visible regularly at ward level during the day and night, by means of some rota system? Why is it not possible for patients and front-line staff to see that senior managers really do have the interests of the patients as their top priority? That may seem mere window-dressing, but if senior managers walked the 'shop floor' (in the manner of a hotel's general manager) it would make a big difference to attitudes at ward level. I can hear cries of protest from healthcare managers telling me they already do much of this, in addition to the vast amount of time they spend strategising, prioritising, planning and controlling. If that is the case I congratulate them, but the practice is not universal.

Common experience?

This chapter started life as a lengthy account of my experiences as a patient, entitled *Being Patient*. I sent personal and confidential copies of my first draft to a selection of people I knew quite well, including: senior civil servants; senior representatives of an employers' body, a national patient representative, a public policy academic, a health service commentator and writer, a hospital non-executive director, two former health service managers and others. Their judgement could be trusted and I wanted to know whether my account would be helpful to clinicians, managers and patients and if I was being fair. Each and every one of my contacts (except for one who didn't reply) found *Being Patient* a great help and all encouraged me to have it published. Their comments included:

> *I think 'Being Patient' is superb. I have read it twice and thought about it a lot. It is uncomfortable reading as it touches on what the NHS should be doing well and consistently as a matter of basic routine.*

> *I do not think this is merely a personal and cathartic exercise . . . the content is of general relevance and interest to anyone working for or receiving treatment from the NHS.*

> *You keep your eyes on the key issues. And you write with conviction and power. I think without any doubt at all you should offer the piece to . . . Ministers and managers. I am so glad you wrote the piece. It is important. It must be published. Thank you very much indeed for sharing it with me.*

> *Wonderful. It was just a wonderful read. Brilliant. I loved it – literate, interesting, real, gripping.*

Encouraged by their comments, I issued *Being Patient* privately to various policy makers, clinicians, managers and regulators. The response was mixed: some welcomed it and began using it in training programmes or for hospital board briefings, some invited me to meetings to discuss its application, and some were deafening in their silence and lack of acknowledgement. I can understand their reticence and their unspoken comments might have included: *'Isn't he grateful we saved his life, twice?'; 'His criticisms are unfair'; 'His experiences aren't typical'; 'That's how it used to be but things have changed now'; 'He's causing trouble';* and such like. I remind you that I sent *Being Patient* only to people I had known for many years.

In 2009, I had the opportunity to present my thoughts in a 60-minute seminar at the European Healthcare Management Association annual conference, in Innsbruck.[1] The audience of 60–70 people consisted of clinicians, managers, academics, policy makers and others from a dozen or so countries and unsurprisingly (or should that be surprisingly?) they recognised what I had to say as all-too-familiar features of many healthcare systems. Although I address in this chapter ways in which these deficient variations should be tackled, the widespread acknowledgement of the existence of such acts of commission and omission suggests to me that further research needs to be undertaken to identify causes and solutions, or reasons and remedies.

I do not believe that my experiences are a one-off and my membership of the Institute for Healthcare Improvement,[2] featuring the pioneering work of Don Berwick and others on quality of healthcare and much else, convinces me that my experiences are merely representative of what happens all too frequently. Often, other patients are unable to articulate their thoughts in a way that will get things changed, or they do not know how to go about it, or they are too ill or just too grateful to follow up their experience with a letter to the hospital management. Therefore, my thoughts are made available for the benefit of all those who have spoken to me and for patients everywhere who believe that although the health services are wonderful, they could be even better.

Being patient focused

This, if you like, is my patient's charter for managers, written with confidence that the lives of patients would be much better if only you could achieve these measures.

1 Work to eradicate the curse of variation

Commit yourself to doing everything you can to eradicate – or at the very least to achieve the minimum amount of – unacceptable and unplanned variation. You need to be certain of those areas in your hospital services that are subject to variation, know the reasons for the variation, and then you need to introduce effective actions, including regular checks and helpful feedback, to ensure that your actions have had the required effect. In the words of the rather overworked cliché, this is not rocket science. It is good old-fashioned management and yet it is not being undertaken across all of healthcare.

2 Introduce effective information systems

This is not a plea to invest millions of pounds in a sophisticated IT system. I really am not making a point about the vehicle you choose to achieve these effective information systems: if quill pens and clerks with starched collars work for you, then so be it! The point I make is that it really beggars belief if in this day and age effective information systems are unavailable.

3 Ensure all services are fully connected

Believe me, your systems really do not work as efficiently as you have been led to believe. Why not go out and discover how the 'white spaces' on your charts might contain a variety of practices unknown to senior management. How about looking at a hospital, or a department within a hospital, where they have already addressed these issues and where they have already successfully joined up patient services. I assure you these places are a joy for patients.

4 Contribute to the patient–clinician relationship

I realise this is a difficult area, as it might be interpreted as undermining the professional standing of the clinician. Tread carefully if you must, but please do not neglect to make a contribution in this important area.

Whilst the overall majority of clinicians, and other front-line staff, are excellent in terms of their relationship with patients, there is a small but significant minority who lack some of the basic requirements (to express myself diplomatically).

How effective are your patient questionnaires or satisfaction surveys? Do they really do the job, or are they simply 'happiness sheets' where the patient, so glad to be going home safe and well, just ticks the 'very good' and 'excellent' boxes? If you are genuinely committed to the quality of your services then really you ought to do something to improve this area.

5 Provide effective training and development for your staff

Health services should be congratulated on their longstanding commitment to education, learning, training and development. In each of these four areas it has an enviable track record. However, the challenge is never ending and even more needs to be done.

6 Try to eliminate poor communication

When communication is working well, people hardly notice it, they just take it for granted, but when communication is poor it is usually the source of dissatisfaction and even complaint: *'Why wasn't I told this?' 'Why wasn't this made clear to me?' 'Why didn't you tell me?'*

7 Reflect on your priorities

Managers may wish to adjust some of their priorities. I know many senior healthcare managers and appreciate how sincere they are about health services, but I also know the vast amounts of time they spend on work that appears to have only a passing relevance to the immediate and future direct needs of patients. Sometimes, this work is inevitable and is encouraged by the various responses they have to give Government initiatives, but at other times the amount of senior management work on producing strategies, policies, plans and initiatives (and then another raft of strategies, policies, plans and initiatives) can be reduced, or even avoided completely. It would be much better, in the humble opinion of this patient, if senior managers committed themselves more to the removal of as much unacceptable variation as possible.

CONCLUSION

My words should not be interpreted as an attack or general complaint about the state of services – that would be untrue and unfair. These words represent solely the view from my 'bed and bath' and it is my hope that individual healthcare managers and clinicians will respond positively to such comments and challenges.

REFERENCES

1 My PowerPoint™-based presentation, *Being Patient: communication and its impact on innovation through the eyes of a patient (and former healthcare senior manager)*, is available on the EHMA website at www.ehma.org/?q=node/221

   A fuller version of the paper is scheduled for publication in the *Journal of Management and Marketing in Healthcare*, January 2010.

2 Institute for Healthcare Improvement – *see* www.ihi.org/ihi. Membership is free.

CHAPTER 7

Building effective organisations:
the lesson of Nigel the bricklayer

Nine summers ago, I spent far too much time at home convalescing after a stay at one of the NHS's finest hospitals. As I walked tentatively outside the house for the first time, I was fascinated to see a wall being built in my neighbour's garden. Each day, with commendable regularity and dedication, the bricklayer would work from early morning to early evening building his splendid garden wall, supported by vast quantities of tea and the delights of Radio 1. For the first few days I had been puzzled about what he was building. There was little to be seen, as he spent hours preparing the foundations, but after a day or so the first few bricks appeared above ground level.

I was fascinated by the progress he made and full of admiration for his skill. I could not build a wall in a month of Sundays, or at least not one that would stand the force of even a gentle breeze. It made me feel quite inadequate, and I remembered reading a volume of Churchill's autobiography in which he described retreating from the political scene to weekends of peace and tranquillity at Chartwell and the work of rebuilding his garden wall.

As the days went by the wall began to 'grow', and each step in the process seemed to require vast amounts of sweat, bricks, cement, pieces of string, spirit levels, trowels, tea, music and numerous inspections of his work from different perspectives. It became a work of art for him and a source of admiration for me.

During the week I got to know Nigel. At first it was no more than a nod of the head as I went for another recuperative walk in the garden. He was busy and a little shy (as I found out later), and I found it difficult to say anything significant about his wall. Everything I thought of sounded so obvious and trite. After a few days we started talking – about the weather, football and, finally, the wonderful wall. He found it very surprising that anyone could be so impressed by something he could do almost with his eyes shut – building walls is what Nigel did best.

When I asked him to explain to me how he built a wall, an expression close to suspicion passed across his face. It was quite clear that he had never been asked such a stupid question in his whole life. At first he was hesitant, but after some appreciative nods from me, and questions that confirmed my genuine interest, he got into his stride. Nigel was not the most talkative of individuals, and if he had built his wall in the order that he described the steps then I doubt if it would have stood for any longer than one built by me. But what he told me amazed me. Without realising it, Nigel had given me a perfect metaphor for the development of most healthcare organisations. His method of wall building took place in four stages, but these four stages had a much richer, deeper meaning for me.

NIGEL'S PRINCIPLES

He explained that it was essential to start with the foundations. This stage was the hardest part of the job – a lot of shovelling and digging – but it was certainly the most important part. It was also the only part of the job where people could not see what had been done, but if it was not done properly, the wall would almost certainly fall down. I wondered how he knew how deep to dig the foundations, and I thought it likely that there was a formula to guide him – something like foundation = depth × ½ length × height ÷ 2 – but Nigel was amused by the very thought of this suggestion. 'No, no', he said, 'you just keep on digging down until you hit something hard!' I was surprised by his answer, but I saw the application of the principle immediately.

'Once you've done your foundations, you start building the wall', he volunteered, obviously warming to his task of instructing an imbecile. 'Can you start building anywhere?' I asked him. 'Oh yes, as long as it's in a corner', he responded. He then explained to me that making sure that the cornerstones were in place was critical to the strength of the wall. It was also essential to make sure that when the other bricks were put in place they were level with the corners, so it was important to check the level and height of the bricks, layer by layer, against the level of the corners. That is why he used the spirit level regularly and why the piece of string gave him 'his level'. Again, I saw immediately how Nigel's principle could be applied to healthcare organisations.

The next thing to puzzle me was why he repeatedly broke a brick in half and inserted it in the wall to create a regular pattern of T-shapes, one on top of the other. This, he told me, was to give the wall maximum strength. Here, warming to his subject even more, he volunteered the fact that this broken brick was called a bonding brick, and that typically there were four styles that could be used in bricklaying – the stretcher, the English garden wall, the old English garden, and the Flemish. How something that had been broken could be turned into a source of strength called out to me about a fundamental principle of life in healthcare organisations.

He explained the fourth stage: 'After that it's just the hard graft of filling up all the gaps with layer after layer of bricks.'

And there you have it – Nigel's four-stage method of building a garden wall. As you will appreciate, any deficiency in my record of this technique is due entirely to my limited memory and understanding of what he said. It is not a reflection of his skill as a bricklayer. For me the matter had little to do with the physical task of building a wall – for Nigel, unknown to him, had given me four wonderful principles to apply to individuals and healthcare organisations as they seek to develop themselves. In subsequent years I have used the Nigel the Bricklayer approach to building health service organisations and developing people on many occasions, and it has always been seen as an effective and enjoyable metaphor.

As I ended my conversation with Nigel I made a tactical error. I explained to him that what he had told me was so interesting and helpful that I was sure I could turn it into an article to help in the work I did, when I was not walking around the garden. That did it. He'd never met anyone like me before – I couldn't even build a garden wall, yet I was prepared to write about it and use what he had told me to help others.

Nigel the Bricklayer

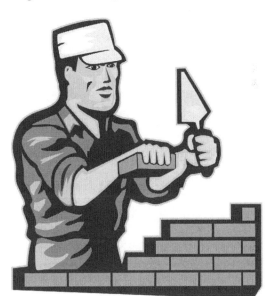

- Foundations

- Cornerstones

- Bonding brick

- Hard work

FOUR ORGANISATIONAL PRINCIPLES
Strong foundations

Nigel's *first principle* is that if you want to build anything that is going to last, you must have a strong foundation. Without a strong foundation your efforts will ultimately prove to be in vain, and what you have tried to construct, or perhaps have already constructed, will eventually come crashing down around you.

I have seen, time after time, what happens when this principle is not adhered to. Along comes an individual and they're so full of themselves. They are going to transform everything. Never mind careful analysis of the key issues before systematically weighing up the options and coming to a considered judgement. They claim to know the answers from the start, and they usually justify their lack of groundwork with words like *intuition* and *judgement*, and even with being *entrepreneurial*. I happen to believe in all three of these concepts and see them as critical to the successful development of any organisation, but with these individuals they are often no more than words they have learned to spout like some form of mantra. There is such a thing as *intuition*, but it is usually based on years of experience. The same is true of the notion of *judgement*, and I readily accept that it appears to be far more finely tuned in some individuals than in others. And all of us should celebrate the truly *entrepreneurial* character, for without them, including their seemingly inevitable string of failures, the world of healthcare would be a much duller place. But the people I am referring to are not true entrepreneurs – it is merely their cover story to obfuscate the fact that they lack the basic grounding in their area of so-called expertise.

It is essential to have a solid foundation, and there is often no short cut to getting one. Just like Nigel, you may find laying the foundation the hardest part of the job, and often it is invisible when being undertaken – reading, studying, building up experience – but one day the evidence of the work will be evident for all to see. They will see the benefit of your groundwork, and you will certainly experience the benefit of the hours that have been put in. I assume (although I could be wrong) that when a wall is built the foundations will last a lifetime, but it is certainly not the same when building the foundations of a career or a healthcare organisation. These foundations need continual attention; they need to be reinforced; they need to be strengthened – and a lack of attention to these needs will one day catch someone out in a world that is changing rapidly.

Julian Boyd (not his real name) was a perfect example of how this principle works. He was brought in to be chief executive of an NHS organisation that had been struggling with a difficult environment. Superficially, Julian had it all – the sound of his voice, the cut of his suit, his inspirational way of talking and his belief that he could transform the organisation. But the more I watched Julian, the more convinced I and many others became that he represented a triumph of style over substance. To change metaphors and use a horticultural one, Julian was a hothouse plant (a rare orchid, perhaps), and when he was exposed to the heat of healthcare realities it soon became clear that his roots did not go deep enough, and in the intense heat of the sun they just withered away. He could not handle the complexities of healthcare life, with its numerous stakeholders and the seemingly conflicting pressures that they exerted. He was far too committed to the 'vision thing', as he called it, and as such did not see the relative mess being generated in the day-to-day management of the organisation. Above all, he confused the generation of even more strategies with the delivery of the current year's business plan objectives. He left the organisation with more problems than it had had when he started, but his elegance will long be remembered. If he had had better prepared foundations he might have lasted the course.

The 'Julians' of this world are an example – an example of how not to lead a healthcare organisation. Their type of leadership is experienced in all types of organisations, of whatever sector, and there is a far greater understanding of when they can be used to advantage and when they are nothing more than a downright liability. In Chapter 1 on leadership I discussed the type of leader described as *narcissistic* and show the ways in which they can benefit or damage an organisation. There is also a growing interest in what are called *level 5 leaders* (again discussed in the chapter on leadership) and the way in which they bring together professional will and personal humility for the benefit of the organisation. They are the very antithesis of Julian and his style.

Julian was a leader of the category known as the *'veni, vidi, vanished'* variety, unfortunately all too common in healthcare. He *came* and made sure that everyone knew that he was around. He *saw* and made a number of decisions based on his imperfect understanding of the situation. He *vanished* as he possessed the innate ability to jump before he was pushed. Why is it that some healthcare organisations appear to be outwardly mature, yet they become infatuated by the Julians of this world, as if they were no more than some form of adolescent organisation? These organisations can be mature in so many ways, yet they still fall prey to the wooings and clichés of someone like Julian. They are overly impressed by a person from another sector, or someone who is so different from their existing batch of managers, and they apparently forget to undertake the most basic of searches into their backgrounds.

Vision, mission and values

Nigel's *second principle* concerns cornerstones – getting them square, aligning them properly, and making sure that all of the bricks laid subsequently are *true* to the cornerstones. This, in organisation development terms, represents the world of vision, mission and values. These three terms have entered the world of jargon in some organisations and so have been called something different – *purpose* being one of the favourite substitute words – but whatever they are called, they remain an essential component for setting direction. Without a sense of vision and mission, and without a proper set of values, any healthcare organisation (and the individuals within it) will find itself struggling to handle fundamental leadership challenges and thereby run the risk of being torn by dilemmas: 'Should we do this?' 'Is this in keeping with what this trust wants to do?' – not to mention statements that really test the mettle, such as 'But everyone else is doing it!' The world of vision, mission and values is critically important.

Theologians may wish to debate the exact meaning of the verse 'Where there is no vision, the people perish' (Proverbs 29:18), but in the world of leadership of healthcare organisations there is little room for doubt – without a clear vision of the purpose of the trust, etc., there is usually a catastrophe waiting around the corner. The hospital trust will find it difficult to set its priorities and to agree on key strategies, and will inevitably experience chaos as different leaders pursue different priorities. The idea of agreeing on a vision statement (even if it is called something else) means that there can be agreement about the major direction being pursued by the healthcare enterprise.

As Kouzes and Posner[1] have shown, the word *vision* in a vision statement signifies that an organisation wishes to be forward-looking and foresighted, possess a future orientation, have a picture of what could be, connote a standard of excellence and suggest a quality of uniqueness. The organisation wants to say that it has an idea of where it wants to go – it has a route map. Mayo and Lank,[2] in their work on learning strategies, see vision as one of the key mechanisms for providing '. . . a rudder to keep the learning process on course when stresses develop . . .', and they make the eminently sensible point that all vision statements must be shared rather than simply imposed on others. It is clear that there are many benefits when the vision statement is used dynamically, including the motivational advantage of having all personnel pulling in the same direction. Rather dramatically, Mayo and Lank cite the motivational pull of two vision statements: Komatsu's 'Kill Caterpillar' and Fujitsu's 'Beat IBM'.

Other vision statements are less blood-curdling, but they all have the potential to improve the performance and commitment of employees. Examples include 'A personal computer on every desk and in every home' (Microsoft), 'A Coke within arm's reach of everyone on the planet' (Coca-Cola) and, perhaps the most famous of all, John F Kennedy's historic declaration in April 1961 that the United States would 'put a man on the moon by the end of the decade'.[3] Notable others include 'To solve unsolved problems innovatively' (3M) and 'To make people happy' (Walt Disney).[4]

The world of mission statements is clouded by the fact that some organisations refer to their mission statement when, to all intents and purposes, they actually mean what most people regard as the standard definition of a vision statement. Most people regard a vision statement as being a brief description of why the organisation exists, and a mission statement as the description of the principal ways in which the vision will be achieved (but even this simple differentiation is likely to raise issues of disagreement). Some will refer to the *mission* of Federal Express as being 'Absolutely, Positively, Overnight',[5] when my definition would see that as a vision statement; and others cite the St Paul's Cathedral vision statement 'To proclaim the Christian gospel according to the practices and traditions of the Church of England and, in an environment of excellence and beauty, to uplift the minds of men, women, and children to things of the spirit',[6] when I regard that to be more of a mission statement.

While not wanting to become bogged down with semantics, many organisational writers use a dated example from the world of health to illustrate the classic mission statement:

> Glaxo is an integrated research-based group of companies whose corporate purpose is to create, discover, develop, manufacture and market throughout the world safe, effective medicines of the highest quality which will bring benefits to patients through improved longevity and quality of life, and to society through economic value.[7]

BOX 7.1 The house illustration

> Over the years I have worked with some truly inspiring people. One of the best was Dame Rennie Fritchie. In addition to holding various public appointments, Rennie had her own consultancy. When we collaborated on a conference for health service trusts that were about to merge, Rennie introduced them to her house analogy to illustrate the different aspects of corporate life. In a chapter based on the activities of a bricklayer, Rennie's house-building analogy seems especially apposite.

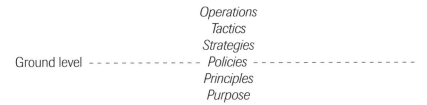

Her *purpose* and *principles* correspond to my *vision, mission* and *values*, and the way in which they relate to the remaining activities of the organisation is demonstrated powerfully by this illustration.

If the vision statement sets out what the healthcare organisation wants to *be*, and the mission statement identifies the steps that have to be taken in order to achieve that vision, then the values statement explains how the organisation will act in its pursuit of its goals. They are the 'organisation's essential and enduring tenets, a small set of guiding principles, which are never compromised for financial gain or short-term expediency'.[8] They are 'what we stand for'.

Examples of corporate values are numerous, and include Merck's unequivocal excellence in all aspects of the company, Nordstrom's service to the customer above all else and Walt Disney's fanatical attention to consistency and detail.[9]

It is all too easy to be cynical about the utility of values, but more and more healthcare organisations are seeing them as an essential part of their way of life. They help to energise staff and gain their commitment, and values can be useful when managing change and in seeing a management or clinical team through various crises. If I had been writing this paragraph a few years earlier, I would have felt the need to develop further my argument on the importance of values. I would have become an apologist for values (and their close cousins – ethics and principles), but there is little need to do that now, thanks to the effort of some major global companies and international financial consultancies. Anyone with a modicum of common sense will realise that values, applied sincerely and consistently, are a critical component of organisational life. The moment for values has arrived for all organisations, and in healthcare they have always been a readily accepted basis for managerial practice.

However, those values have to be meaningful and have to be seen by employees to be sensible, ideally something that they have helped to develop, and a genuine description of the ethos of practice. When I attended a seminar in the London headquarters of a well-known and successful major British company, they had on the wall of their impressive entrance hall two screens that showed an electronic display of their values – a very impressive display and one which showed the visitor that here was an organisation clear about its values. Over dinner, I asked two of their senior managers about the values display and was told, in hushed tones, that they had been developed recently by the board, and that they had been developed within the confines of the boardroom. The board had been advised by a number of senior executives not to publish them before an extensive consultation exercise had been initiated, but they refused. They were apparently very proud of their work on developing a values statement, especially one that had been based on an acronym, and the electronic values were greeted with more than a degree of bemusement by the very people who had to make them work.

Individual managers, if they belong to professional bodies such as the Institute of Healthcare Management, will be all too familiar with the way in which values are informing the plethora of codes of practice emerging to cover managerial activities. Never has there been such a clear need to demonstrate that one's actions are governed by some set of principles and standards, and chief executives and executive directors, especially, are feeling the wind of change as advances are being made to ensure the highest standards of corporate governance.

Many healthcare organisations have had in place statements of vision, mission and values for many years, but have found that their statements no longer reflect the realities of life in the twenty-first century. This is despite the rhetoric that claims vision and values should be sustained irrespective of time – they are, or should be, timeless. But life is never that simple, and most healthcare organisations will find that there comes a time when everything needs to be reviewed. Sull[10] illustrates this point in his inspiring article 'Why Good Companies Go Bad', and shows that an organisation's decline may be associated with strategies that have become 'blinders', processes becoming routines, relationships becoming shackles and, significantly, values becoming dogmas that no longer motivate but instead cause active inertia.

Brokenness and humility

The *third principle* was not Nigel's at all, or at least it was not a point that he made directly. When he spoke about how the use of a broken brick added strength to the wall, the general principle for healthcare organisations became very clear. The third principle is that brokenness and humility will add strength to any individual and to any organisation. It may not be very fashionable to talk in this way about the merits of brokenness and humility, as it seems to fly in the face of far more positive-sounding concepts such as wholeness and pride. So let me explain what I mean by these concepts.

The first thing to emphasise is that there is absolutely nothing wrong with concepts such as *wholeness* and *pride*. Wholeness is a good thing – it implies unity, something that is not damaged or deprived of any part, and of course it conjures up links to the word 'wholesome'. Pride in one's achievements is also commendable, as is pride in one's work. Pride becomes a problem when it is used as a divisive factor, or to hurt someone else through acts that suggest a superior position in life.

However, *brokenness* and *humility* are also important characteristics and they should not be seen as mutually exclusive with regard to the concepts of wholeness and pride. They can exist alongside one another. Anyone who has held a senior position in healthcare will know that there are many trials and tribulations to be experienced during a career – for example, the plan that did not go through as expected; the difficult group of people you were asked to manage; or the project where, quite frankly, you screwed up. When these things happen it is possible for the individual and the organisation to respond in one of two ways. The problems can either destroy the individual or they can make him or her wiser and more mature, a person whose judgement has improved immeasurably. Some people, when faced with supposedly overwhelming challenges such as these, will crawl away and allow their careers to die, or else their organisations, revealing an alarming case of myopia, will do it on their behalf. What a waste this is. If the individual is a competent and committed person who just happened to make a mistake, then he or she should be helped to overcome the experience, to learn from it and to emerge from it as a stronger individual (unless it was a truly catastrophic mistake). Unfortunately, such an approach is alien to some healthcare organisations, and their prevailing culture suggests that it is a case of 'one mistake and you're out'. What a waste of talent this is. Most people can benefit substantially from the experience of having been a 'broken brick', and as stronger and wiser individuals they can be used to add strength to the organisation. One day I shall run a conference called 'The three biggest mistakes I made and what I learned from them'. It should be a sell-out and encourage people to be honest about their careers instead of pretending that mistakes do not happen. Such a conference would also help to stop this ridiculous practice of sweeping errors under the carpet. It is much better, as a general rule, to have errors out in the open so that others can learn from them. There should be a system whereby these experiences can be shared with younger managers in the hope that they will not make the same mistakes, and to show them that they work for an organisation in which real learning, from all kinds of source, takes place. All similar experiences should become a part of the learning system that operates within healthcare organisations.

Humility is similar. I have met a large number of people, from many different walks of life, who have been hugely successful in their profession. They may have been successful in their careers, or in education, or in the arts, but one thing has typified them by and large – the more successful they were, the more self-effacing they had become. The opposite is also true. This is not a universal principle, and I know that there are some successful people who do not make for pleasant company, but my general observation holds true. The more successful the person, the more humble they are likely to be, and the less successful the person, the more likely they are to be a loudmouth whose companionship is not something to relish. It seems to be a general law of life that the more one knows about the multi-dimensional world of healthcare organisations, and of life in general, the more one realises the true extent of personal knowledge – everyone has a lot to be humble about!

Without humility a person will never be a true learner. To start with they will not have enough self-awareness – the ability to take a truly dispassionate look at themselves – and they will think that penetrative, insightful points are always being made about someone else and never about them. They will certainly not be over-keen on hearing what others think about a particular situation, and they will lose the benefit of valuable insights from others. Typically they will be poor listeners – they are far too busy talking – and will therefore lose the benefits that flow from being open to new ideas from others.

Hard work

The *fourth principle* is hard work. 'Filling the gaps' and 'layer after layer of bricks' is what Nigel would call it. It should come as no surprise to hear that there is no substitute for hard work. Wherever I go I discover that successful people work hard. There is absolutely no substitute for being dedicated and translating that dedication into blood, sweat and tears. The principle applies equally to those who wish to become successful bricklayers and to those who want to run a successful healthcare organisation or department.

There are places to visit, people to see, meetings to attend, documents to read, papers to prepare, problems to deal with, agreements to make, and all of it takes time and effort. It just has to be done. Most successful people will agree with the well-known golfing maxim, 'The more I practise the luckier I get'. It is the same with work, and the greater the effort put into the work the greater the reward obtained from it. There really are no alternatives to hard work.

But working hard is not the same as being trapped in a long-hours culture. Far too many people sacrifice all other parts of their life in pursuit of a successful career. Their partner and children trail a poor second to the possibility of enhancement at work. How sad this is. What a tragedy this is. Some people are even prepared to put their physical and emotional health on the line and end up reliant on the comfort of some form of stimulant (ranging from litres of coffee to many stronger items) in an attempt (and usually a vain one) to keep things going and to keep climbing the corporate ladder.

In stark contrast, there are the really clever people who have figured out how to work hard without sacrificing all other parts of their life and health. Or they have discovered how to create a better balance between what they want from work and from the rest of their life. They know how to work effectively, to 'work smart', to manage their time and to achieve something approaching a work–life balance. They know the advantages of using the revolution in information technology to their advantage, the joy of home working (how many hours are wasted each day by commuters fighting to get into work?), and many other devices that are available when they take the effort to find out about them.

There is much to be gained from a careful analysis of one's work and from facing up to the hours, and even days, that can be wasted by needless or ineffective work in a week. Think of those pointless meetings you have attended, when even after the meeting you were not too sure of its real purpose; or those journeys you have undertaken when a reasonably priced video-conferencing system would have saved hours in the car, train or plane; or those papers you have written when a face-to-face meeting or phone call would have had the same result. Think of the healthcare organisation you are in where there isn't a clearly thought-out strategy; or the department that frequently does not have the time to do things right the first time, but always finds time (usually your time) to remedy the problem. I could go on, but I am sure the message is clear – hard work must be effective work. A radical analysis of the time spent on various activities in a week will always pay dividends.

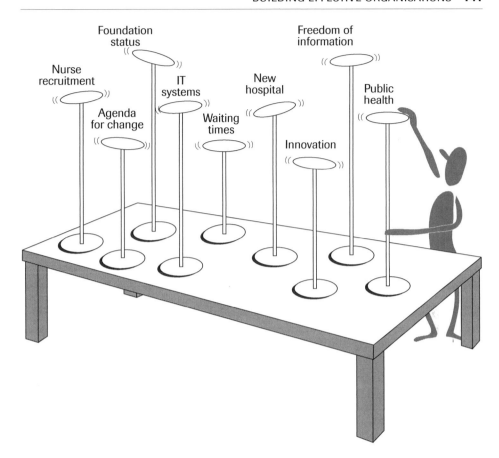

FIGURE 7.1 Management 'plate spinning'

FROM THEORY TO PRACTICE

For many years the idea of improvisation has fascinated me. I was first introduced to the subject by a cousin of mine who worked as a director in a provincial
theatre. The actors, all of whom were experienced individuals, would stage plays
without the benefit of a detailed script, and from an outline of the general direction of the story they would allow the play to follow the energy they obtained
from the audience. No doubt there was also an element of individual actors
thinking they might like to experiment, or even cause 'trouble' for one of their
colleagues, by asking them to respond to an implausible developing plot. My
cousin was a great believer in the improvisation genre, and would regale me with
stories of how successful and energising such an approach had proved.

The same is true of music. There is a world of difference between an orchestra
with a score in front of it and the discipline of the various parts of the orchestra,
and the techniques occasionally employed by a jazz quartet when they decide
to 'let it all hang out'. As I am typing these words I am listening to Bach's *Mass
in B Minor* (does that say something about my state of mind?), and I am grateful for a disciplined orchestra following the score and the direction of Herbert
von Karajan. Later today, I might listen to one of the jazz greats and admire

their ability to seemingly 'make it up as they go along'. Both forms of music are inspiring.

What is obvious, both on the stage and in the concert hall, is that the actors and musicians – whether they are following a script or a score, or improvising – are consummate professionals who are capable of performing through both mediums, and that each medium demands expertise, discipline and considerable practice. The formal set-piece display and the less formal improvised approach both require just as much practice and professionalism. It is merely that the manifestation of this expertise looks and sounds different and can provoke different responses in the audience.

It may seem strange to suggest that similar approaches to set scores and improvisation should be displayed in healthcare organisations, but that is surely a healthy way to view the need for leaders at times to perform in accordance with laid down procedures, and at other times, as needs demand, to utilise their vast experience and professionalism and engage in the equivalent of improvisation – to do the equivalent of 'making it up as they go along'. There are many examples of healthcare organisations that become hidebound through being fixated on procedure, and it would do them the world of good to 'loosen up' and improvise their way through a management challenge. Similarly, there are some healthcare organisations that are never happier than when improvising, and that 'sail far too close to the wind' of bad practice, through their avoidance of formalised procedures and adherence to sensible, laid-down management systems. The healthy position, surely, is to know when to be formal (to engage in planning, procedures and tight governance systems) and when it is best to 'hang loose' (and allow the creative juices to flow).

I was intrigued to be sent an article entitled 'The Improvising Organisation: where planning meets opportunity',[11] in which four writers make much the same point. With persuasive arguments they contend that:

> What distinguishes the best companies from all others is a superior ability to adapt to and capitalize on a rapidly changing and often unpredictable environment. Conversely, many large companies have fallen on hard times because they have been unable to innovate and renew themselves . . . These companies . . . err by assuming that the business environment is knowable and therefore largely predictable . . . The answer is to augment traditional planning with *improvisation techniques used in music and theatre.* (My italics.)

They go on to argue that:

> no matter how many times managers have been told by the likes of Henry Mintzberg and Tom Peters that they cannot plan their way into the future, they retain a powerful corporate planning and control mind-set. Their overriding assumptions about the future business environment remain: it is largely predictable, and control of the firm's performance in that environment is possible.

What the authors show is that formal approaches and the less formal, but certainly not informal (as that suggests a certain lackadaisicalness), approach to management are both legitimate. The successful healthcare organisations know when to employ which approach, and both approaches require disciplined, experienced and dedicated managers. The difference is that different circumstances require different approaches, and the wise healthcare management team knows when to act appropriately.

Which brings me back to the principles we learned from Nigel the bricklayer. If leaders wish to depart from the script or score, if they wish to be more spontaneous, and if they want to improvise their response to various challenges, it is essential that their actions should be based on solid foundations: a clear set of espoused and practised values, a learning system that is open to the ideas of others, and on a large amount of humility – and sheer hard work. Without that assurance, the improvised or intuitive response is just plain foolishness – a knee-jerk reaction rather than one based on years of hard work, experience and judgement. A successful healthcare organisation can only engage in what appears to be 'making it up as we go along' when the leaders and managers running it are certain that their foundations are solid, they are open to one another, they know that their colleagues will function in a way that is consistent with their values, and everyone is prepared to roll up their sleeves and make sure that the thing works.

I assert this with such confidence because I have seen it work. Between 1995 and 2001 I was the Chief Executive of the National Health Service Staff College Wales. This virtual college was established in order to provide a leadership and learning development facility for the health service and to contribute to the change management agenda. It soon spread its wings and became a major focus for management research activity, educational programmes and some health service development initiatives. When the college started life in 1995, it had five staff, which included two administrative staff, and a small annual budget. By 2001, when I left, it had almost 60 staff and a multi-million-pound budget. Without doubt much of the success was down to the quality of its staff, the fact that it delivered valued and relevant work, and no doubt there was an element of luck in being in the right place at the right time. But I believe that the most significant factor in its success was that it adhered to the four principles enunciated in this chapter. It had people with solid and deep foundations developed over years of experience – they had a solid track record. The value system was clear and was lived out in all of the activities, thereby reducing the time-consuming administrative chores that stultify the growth of many organisations. There was a team consisting of members who tried to be honest with one another and spent time learning from successes and (many) failures. And finally there was a group of people who were so enthused by what they did that they found work to be a pleasant activity and so strove to make it a success. Nigel's principles are not just theory – they work.

Key actions

1 Take well-thought-out steps to ensure that the foundation of your career is solid. You should be willing to discuss your qualifications, experience and development plan with a coach or management development adviser.

2 Be clear about the values of your organisation and make sure, wherever possible, that they are congruent with your personal values. You should be able to explain, in simple terms, what you and your organisation are trying to achieve.

3 Encourage individuals to learn from both success and failure and practise management as a humble person rather than as a proud one.

4 No doubt you work hard – everyone in healthcare does that – but it is important to commit yourself to a 'work–life' balance. Your family needs you and you need them.

REFERENCES

1 Kouzes JM and Posner BZ (1995) *The Leadership Challenge*. Jossey-Bass, San Francisco, CA.

2 Mayo A and Lank E (1994) *The Power of Learning*. Chartered Institute of Personnel and Development, London.

3 Garratt B (1996) *The Fish Rots from the Head*. HarperCollins Business, London.

4 Collins C and Porras J (1991, 1992, 1995–98). *Harvard Business Review on Change*. Harvard Business School Press, Boston, MA.

5 Wickens PD (1995) *The Ascendant Organisation*. Palgrave Macmillan, Basingstoke.

6 Pasternack B and Viscio A (1999) *The Centerless Corporation*. Booz, Allen, Hamilton, McLean, VA.

7 Garratt B (1996) *The Fish Rots from the Head*. HarperCollins Business, London.

8 *Bulletpoint*. Issue 83 (July/August 2001); www.bulletpoint.com

9 Collins C and Porras J (1991, 1992, 1995–98). *Harvard Business Review on Change*. Harvard Business School Press, Boston, MA.

10 Sull DN (2002) Why good companies go bad. In: *Harvard Business Review on Culture and Change*. Harvard Business School Press, Boston, MA.

11 Crossan MM, White RE, Lane HW, *et al.* (1996) The improvising organisation: where planning meets opportunity. *Organiz Dynamics*. 24(4): 20.

CHAPTER 8

Getting to the very heart
of the matter

In the folklore of the Middle East, the story is told about a man named Nasrudin, who was searching for something on the ground. A friend came by and asked 'What have you lost, Nasrudin?'

'My key,' said Nasrudin.

So the friend went down on his knees, too, and they both looked for it. After a time, the friend asked: 'Where exactly did you drop it?'

'In my house,' answered Nasrudin.

'Then why are you looking here, Nasrudin?'

'There is more light here than inside my own house', replied Nasrudin.[1]

The only thing I know about Sufism is that it is based on the teachings of a pantheistic Mohammedan mystic and that it has a seemingly endless raft of stories to illustrate particular principles. Not exactly an encyclopaedic knowledge on my part, I admit, but the above story is a perfect metaphor for what I want to say about getting to the very heart of the matter.

Please spend a minute or two thinking about the story of Nasrudin. Picture the story in your mind and see if you can move your thinking from a position where you might have reacted initially by saying 'What a stupid thing to do!' to a position where you might say to yourself 'What a profound story'. It is easy to dismiss Nasrudin as foolish: 'Can you imagine losing something in your house and then spending your time looking for it outside the house? Not even a relaxing 20 minutes in the sun would make me do that.' Think for a moment. Are there times when you do exactly the same thing? Not with a house key you may have misplaced, but perhaps with aspects of your everyday work. Are there things in your healthcare setting that have been lost – not so much a key or a computer disk, but something significant such as the loyalty of your staff or the performance of your department – and instead of looking in the place where it was probably lost you start looking *outside the house*? There is 'more light' there, or perhaps it is just that it is more comfortable, as it avoids the need to ask some very important and searching questions.

At this point, those who have read the previous paragraph and given it some thought are likely to fall into two camps. The first are those who are beginning to connect with the point I am making, or may even be ahead of me. The second camp are thinking to themselves, 'What on earth is he getting at?' If you fall into the second camp, please read the story of Nasrudin again and think about your own healthcare work. If you still cannot make head or tail of what I am suggesting, please stay with this chapter a little longer, in the hope that all may become clear before too long. If it really is proving quite impossible to remain with this line of thought, please go to the next chapter where there will be no more of this 'touchy-feely' stuff. For those of you who are still with me – thank you, and let us think more about people in our healthcare organisations who might resemble Nasrudin in the way in which they behave.

DEALING WITH PROBLEM ISSUES

Many people see a problem in their healthcare organisation – it may well be to do with performance, or patient care, or the morale of their staff – and the temptation to do something, something tangible, is almost overwhelming:

> There is a problem in my department and I am the one in charge, so I've got to do something about it. Action. Clear action. I must show that I am doing something about the problem. I can't leave this problem to fester. It will get worse and then it will be even harder to solve. What can I do? I must be proactive. I must show I am managing the problem.
>
> And without too much time for reflection, they plunge into management action. It may not solve the problem, but at least they can be seen to be doing something about it.

In these organisations, and at most levels of management, action in response to the problem is put in place, and of course something will begin to happen. The action might not be undertaken as a result of a careful analysis of the underlying causes of the problem – an evidence-based approach, to use the jargon – as there has been no time for such an approach, and to commission evidence gathering might give the appearance to others (especially one's boss) of dithering, of not knowing what to do, of indecision. Such problems call for management action, not evidence gathering! The fact that the all-action managers once read a management theorist who showed that 'today's problems come from yesterday's solutions'[2] or who warned of the dangers of 'symptomatic solutions to systemic problems' is immaterial – it seemed to make sense then and squared with their experience of managerial life, but now it is different. Something has to be done. And so, like Nasrudin in the story above, the managers embark on their course of action. They are operating where they believe there is plenty of light. It might not be where they lost the precious article – the team's performance, or patient care or staff morale – but this is where they think they are likely to find the answer. This is where 'their light' is, or so they think, and this is where they can show best of all that they are taking action.

From my experience, if the challenge being addressed is a major issue then it is likely that this rush into action will take one or more of three forms:

1 there will be a reorganisation of the way things are done, and this will probably involve some form of restructuring of the healthcare organisation *and/or*

2 it will lead to the introduction of some new concept into the organisation based on the latest thinking of some management guru *and/or*

3 there will be a new policy or strategy, described as part of a strategic management response, to meet the need that has arisen in the organisation.

DEALING WITH CAUSES: THE REAL ISSUES

Before I deal with each of these points in turn, I must deal with the hint of cynicism that has found its way into my comments. These three approaches are true of all types of organisation, and should not be seen as peculiar to the health sector. Nor should the three points be interpreted as a criticism of the health service – I am one of its greatest supporters. Also, I am not opposed to reorganising or restructuring an organisation. There are times when it is absolutely essential and the 'proof of the pudding' is the success resulting from such action. Nor am I against some of the new concepts – what critics may call the latest fads – which have been introduced into management, especially over the last 20 years. I have used most of them and believe that they have a major role to play in most healthcare organisations. Nor am I against the introduction of new policies and strategies. How could I be when I have introduced such policies myself, when I have seen strategies reap rich rewards for a healthcare organisation, and when world-class experts (theorists and practitioners) have written so influentially on the subject? My objection concerns those times when the three responses (reorganisation, new concepts and new strategies) are used in a similar way to Nasrudin looking for his key. Too many people confuse relentless, breathtaking activity with meaningful action that tackles the genuine underlying issues within the organisation. In other words, there is an abundance of proactive action, but it is action that does not necessarily address the fundamental issues in the healthcare organisation. The action is dealing with the symptoms of the problem but is not getting to the underlying causes, to the root of the problem – it is not 'getting to the very heart of the matter'.

Systems thinkers – those people who understand that organisations are complex interrelated entities and that isolated initiatives can do more harm than good – appreciate the dangers inherent in dealing with the symptoms of a problem rather than with the underlying reasons that caused it in the first place. Most leaders of healthcare organisations have learned the importance of systems thinking – looking for underlying trends and forces for change – as they are only too aware that:

> The pressures to intervene in management systems that are going awry can be overwhelming. Unfortunately, given the linear thinking that predominates in most organisations, interventions usually focus on symptomatic fixes, not underlying causes. This results in only temporary relief, and it tends to create still more pressures later on for further, low-leverage intervention.[3]

THE TEMPTATION OF CHANGING ORGANISATIONAL STRUCTURES

Anyone who has travelled around offices in different organisations, not only healthcare ones, will almost certainly have seen a quotation by someone called Petronius Arbiter (*c.* AD 60), pinned to the office noticeboard:

> I came to learn later in life that we tend to meet any new situation by reorganising; and a wonderful method it can be for creating the illusion of progress while producing confusion, inefficiency and demoralisation.

Petronius Arbiter lived under the reign of Nero and is mentioned by writers such as Pliny the Elder and Tacitus, although it is not always entirely clear whether he was the author of all the sayings attributed to him. What is clear is that he appears to be one of the most quoted members of the school of ancient organisational philosophers. Even though no such school existed, the retrospective collection of quotes such as these, from a range of Greek philosophers, gives the impression that Athens had a thriving business school long before the birth of Christ!

The Petronius Arbiter poster reveals that these employees, in what appears to be an act of defiance and yet at the same time an act of resigned acquiescence to the latest in a line of reorganisation proposals, find considerable solace in his words. The words might even serve as a source of finger pointing at those senior managers who change organisational structures far too often and without the support of the workforce. As far as the employees are concerned, the organisation's senior management are restructuring for the umpteenth time and yet again, as happened the last time and every previous reorganisation before that, great benefits for the provision of healthcare and its staff are being promised. The proposals claim major cost savings, improvements to the way in which the organisation deals with its patients, and general improvements in the way in which everyday activity is conducted.

The suggestion made by management is that everything will be noticeably better, but the person who placed the Petronius Arbiter quotation on the noticeboard sees things differently. There will be changes. The organisation may be centred around patient services rather than geographical territories; certain new ideas or strategies may be introduced; one or two faces may even appear, but despite these changes eventually, as night follows day, life will go on much the same as before. Those driving through the organisational change programme may interpret such attitudes as unjustifiable cynicism, but those who have experienced the various ways in which the organisation has been organised previously will regard their view as no more than realism based on experience of life in their hospital. At the very least, the reaction of the staff, captured in the Petronius poster, shows that those charged with bringing about change have failed to spend enough time convincing their employees of the genuine need for change. If only these organisations had paid heed to the words of Robert Townsend: 'Reorganisation should be undergone about as often as major surgery. And should be as well planned and as swiftly executed.'[4] If only they had made sure that the proposed changes had been based on hard evidence, that staff had been convinced of the need for change, that the changes would deal with fundamental underlying issues, and that the ideas and genuine concerns of staff had been dealt with in a meaningful way.

ORGANISATIONAL TYPES

Whether or not organisations reorganise, and whether or not the changes are seen as justifiable by the staff, it never fails to surprise me how little imagination some managers put into the type of structures that most organisations introduce. Anyone examining the typical organisation chart will find an all too familiar sight – so many of them follow what is known as the traditional and bureaucratic hierarchical model. In this model (*see* Figure 8.1) one manager oversees the work of four or five others who in turn manage the work of five or six others. The chart has been drawn by someone with the precision of an architect, and unsurprisingly it has a balanced, symmetrical feel to it. There is a sense that this is an organisation that functions extremely efficiently, and that its groups look after departments, and its departments look after units. It is regimented, even militaristic in its appearance, and gives the impression that every activity within the organisation follows a set of formal processes and systems. In the first organisation I worked in I recall being told that as a member of a particular division, especially as I was a humble management trainee, I could only enter into formal communication with a member of another division by following a set of arcane procedures. This involved proceeding up the management hierarchy, with a paper setting out my position, thereby allowing the head of my division to communicate with individuals employed in the other division by means of a memorandum. Thankfully those days have long gone, but the vestiges of them remain in far too many places.

Organisational theorists have a lot to answer for! Even today I am surprised by the number of standard textbooks on organisational theory in which little understanding appears to exist about the variety of potential organisational forms. Most texts introduce the student, even if they are a senior manager, to three basic organisational forms.

There is the traditional hierarchical model, sometimes known as the functional organisation (*see* Figure 8.1).

Then there is the version based on the particular service or 'product' (*see* Figure 8.2) or, just as easily, on a geographical territory.

The concept of the matrix organisation (*see* Figure 8.3) is introduced and the student is made to feel that they are in the presence of leading-edge thinking.

Thankfully, most organisational theorists (and this includes the vast majority of business schools) introduce students and executives to a much wider range of organisational models. The work of Henry Mintzberg, for example, shows the availability of key differences in organisational design 'appropriate to deal with different sets of contingency factors, reflecting variation in the organisation's age, size, technical system and environment'.[5] Mintzberg introduces five types of organisational model, namely the simple structure, machine bureaucracy, professional bureaucracy, the divisionalised and the adhocracy. As you will have gathered by now, my intention in writing this book is not to summarise the content of various textbooks by an array of academics. Their works are

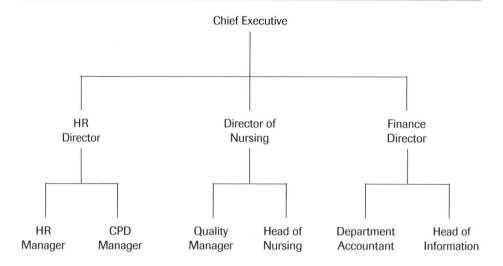

FIGURE 8.1 Traditional hierarchical model

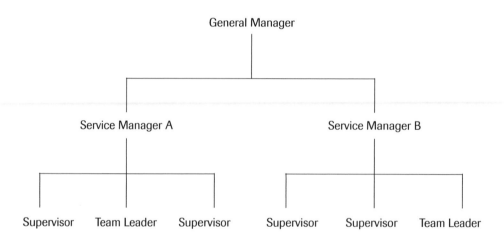

FIGURE 8.2 Typical example of product organisation

accessible and any brief précis of them would be a grave injustice. It is sufficient to refer to Mintzberg's work and to show that various forms of organisations exist and that they are sensitive to the needs of various settings. The experienced healthcare reader will understand this and appreciate that there are far more models available than the traditional hierarchical models so admired in many organisations.

Charles Handy makes a similar point to Mintzberg in his classic work *Gods of Management*.[6] In his inimitable style he uses four gods from Greek mythology to introduce four very different types of organisation (*see* Figure 8.4).

Apollo is the formal role culture much used by traditional organisations.

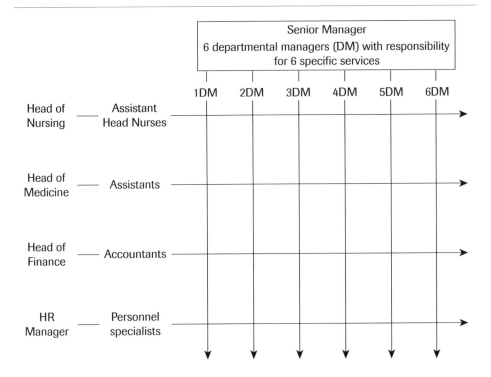

FIGURE 8.3 Typical example of matrix organisation

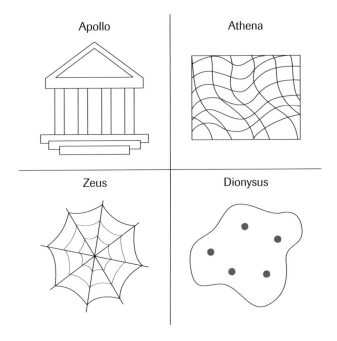

FIGURE 8.4 Charles Handy's 'Gods of Management'
Source: Handy C (1995) *Gods of Management: the changing work of organisations.* Arrow, London.

Work is based around the role and the job to be done, rather than around individuals and the skills and knowledge that they bring to the workplace. *Athena*, on the other hand, is the task culture. With Athena, the solution of problems is the key factor and people are continually drawn into task and project teams. This is matrix management 'gone mad', and is typical of many of the organisations that have been springing up in the 'new economy' of the 1990s and the early part of the twenty-first century. *Zeus* represents the club culture in which all activity derives from and exists around the presence of the 'spider' in the middle of the web. This model is typical of small entrepreneurial entities where contact with the founder – the organisation's inspiring force – is a critical issue. However, anyone who has worked in such an organisation will also know that such a powerful character at the centre of these empires has a magnetic influence on others and is crossed at some peril. Finally, there is *Dionysus* and the existential culture. This organisation is a typical home for barristers, architects and similar professionals. Those who belong to an organisation of this type usually do so grudgingly and only for the benefits that it brings them.

Gareth Morgan[7] takes the design of organisations to a new level and uses metaphors, including the organisation as a machine or as an organism, to help to illustrate the different organisational models. My favourite part of his work, and the one I refer to with clients and colleagues, is his use of a spider plant to show that it is possible to 'grow large whilst remaining small'. The spider plant has the ability to send out shoots that create the image of the 'parent' plant and remain connected to it by the equivalent of an umbilical cord.

He shows that the notion of franchising in retailing can be applied in other contexts, such as large healthcare organisations, and that it is possible to increase the size of an organisation without gargantuan growth in the size of the head office and the bureaucratic procedures that follow. In his version, the organisation must have a clear set of values and operating principles, and 'successful decentralisation depends on the development of good "umbilical cords"'. When I explain this concept to clients they find it an appealing idea but few have the time, or perhaps the courage, to make it a reality in their work environment. It is extremely risky to run a healthcare organisation predominantly on the basis of values, and the production of formalised sets of rules and regulations is a much safer and easier option.

THEORY VS. PRACTICE

During a visit to a healthcare organisation it is a source of fun to compare the formal organisation chart with how things are actually run, as they are rarely the same. Although the organisation chart purports to reflect the organisational arrangements within the healthcare setting, it seldom captures the variety of fluctuations and nuances. If only organisation charts were drawn accurately – they would show the most complicated set of relationships and interrelationships, far too messy for the bureaucratic need to have a piece of paper that suggests order and control.

One organisation that I consulted with regularly, and another in healthcare that I used to run, recognised and celebrated the fact that they had all four of

Charles Handy's 'gods' happily co-existing within their overall structures. Both of these organisations, to ensure that the performance and accountability requirements of their parent body were met, often operated in formal Apollo-mode. To ensure that most of its projects were delivered, the organisation had created a system of teams very similar to Athena-mode. Some of its key clients were Zeus-like in their behaviour, and so the organisation had to respond in that particular style, and some of their own staff, those with an element of prima-donna temperament, worked in a way that would be at home in the Dionysus culture. These two organisations recognised these four styles as a fact of life, and saw them as a virtue rather than a vice, and their acceptance of these different styles has avoided any sense of there being organisational schizophrenia. Although they had a formal organisational chart to satisfy their Apollo-like parent body, their actual chart, if it were ever drawn, would contain the most amazing set of zigzagging lines and unusual relational shapes. When a formal body visited them, they were able to produce an organisation chart showing traditional, hierarchical lines and a well-ordered organisation, but they also adopted variations on that structure on a day-to-day basis. They were thriving organisations because they made a virtue out of their diversity and allowed their staff creative freedom and the ability to respond to the needs of the organisation and its users.

NEW CONCEPTS AND NEW STRATEGIES

Two of the best recent autobiographical management books give dramatic accounts of how Jack Welch[8] transformed General Electric and how Louis Gerstner[9] rescued the commercial reputation of IBM. They are stirring tales, modern classics of managerial adventure. They also offer a detailed insight into the value of introducing appropriate new approaches into an organisation, and of the importance of revising existing strategies and introducing new ones. Without the efforts of Welch, Gerstner and their teams, plus the application of their strategies, it is possible that General Electric and IBM would not be what they are today, and might even have gone to the wall.

My reason for highlighting the sterling efforts of Welch and Gerstner is to make it perfectly clear once again that I am not opposed to new initiatives and strategies aimed at tackling old and new problems. In fact, I am a keen advocate of the majority of new initiatives, and perhaps there were times in my managerial career when I was too great an advocate of new approaches, and a poor reader of the organisational politics as to whether something should be introduced or the best time to introduce it. I have sponsored quality management programmes in healthcare and remain convinced that two of the quality maxims, 'fit for purpose' and 'conformance to standards', have stood the test of time and still have much to offer any healthcare organisation, and indeed the economy at large. I have also welcomed the development of the European Foundation for Quality Management and the work known as Sigma. Benchmarking and business process re-engineering were a joy to sponsor in healthcare. In addition, comparing oneself with leaders in the field and streamlining the way in which management is undertaken in the interest of one's patients or clients made absolute sense then and always will do. I could make similar comments about many other initiatives. The same is true of strategy. I am a firm believer in the importance of developing strategy within an organisation and I realise that, from the perspective of both theory and practice, without strategy most ideas will remain a mere pipedream.

It is not the managers who subscribe to new approaches and new strategies that alarm me, but rather it is those who subscribe to one of the new approaches without having any intention of working with it in a substantial and systematic manner. They are far more interested in being associated with the latest managerial gizmo than with doing something that, over time, will really improve their organisation and its performance. They talk about it, they use all the right jargon, and if there is a chance of putting some symbol on their letterheads that shows their commitment to it, then they are the first in the queue. However, doing something with it, something that will fundamentally alter their organisation, is quite another thing. They are the 'here today, gone tomorrow' brigade. By the time they should be evaluating their last strategy they are far too busy worrying about their next initiative, which will supposedly transform the entire organisation.

MERE MOOSE HEADS!

Gareth Morgan's moose-head cartoon[10] is profound and sums up the approach of the managers I have been describing. In the cartoon he shows a collection of moose heads affixed to a plinth on the boardroom wall, with a number of management initiatives listed below. Each moose head represents an initiative, a programme that has been successfully adopted (although probably not implemented systematically). Quality? Leadership? Re-engineering? Equal opportunities? 'Been there, done that, got the T-shirt', to quote the once popular UK television advert, is their tacit and even outspoken response. They collect these approaches like a child collecting computer games, they sign up for a variety of fanciful initiatives, they drive their staff crazy with yet another new programme, and once they have obtained their 'moose head' they put it on the boardroom plinth and smile at it admiringly once a month. What is worse, they have managed to make their key employees disaffected with any such initiative, and they themselves have become inoculated against the full effect of the initiative's impact. They have experienced a little of its effect, just enough to immunise them against its full effect, and then they move on to look for the next short-term miracle cure for their organisational problems.

Successful healthcare and other organisations that have survived a range of challenging conditions over a long period of time appear to do the very opposite of the quick-fix, short-term approach. In general they choose a new initiative carefully, they try not to make too much of a song and dance about it, they often do not give it a specific title, and they attempt to integrate it into their traditional approach to the management of the organisation. Most importantly, they stick to the chosen approach and work hard to make it a success. They realise that there are few quick-fix solutions to be had, and that most things have to be worked at over a long time. Therefore, the new initiative has more chance of being successful, and if it fails then it will quietly wither away without creating the antagonism that brasher approaches seem to generate.

INTEGRATING INITIATIVES AND STRATEGIES

In the early 1990s, one healthcare organisation (which is now a successful and well-thought-of NHS trust) asked me to work with them on their SIMT programme. When I asked for the acrostic to be explained, they told me that it stood for the *Simultaneous Implementation of Management Techniques*! They intended to roll various new initiatives, such as quality management, benchmarking, re-engineering and much more, into one integrated initiative and then absorb it into everyday management practice. We spent time thinking about it, we examined the common themes of each of the separate programmes and brought together the features of the separate initiatives into one programme – a single SIMT. The theory was impeccable, we had produced the 'simultaneous implementation of management techniques', but in practice the implementation was far more difficult as the already committed front-line managers thought the chief executive had 'bitten off more than they (rather than he) could chew' in one go. I salute them for their efforts, and when I visited them some months and then years later, it was encouraging to see the progress that they had made. In their understated yet comprehensive and methodical way they had achieved much and continued to be one of the leading NHS trusts. They were outwardly rather unassuming, yet they got on with the job and made real progress. There is clear evidence that their continuing progress is due in large part to the mature and sophisticated way in which they tackled and absorbed new opportunities.

Strategy is a similar issue. Everyone accepts that new policies and strategies are essential to a healthcare organisation and its development. However, there are times when the cavalier way in which some managers develop, use and seemingly abuse them makes one wonder whether they really understand this principle at all.

Consider the example of what I call the 'jam tomorrow' user of strategy. They see strategies as an opportunity to promise major transformations in the performance of their department or profession . . . in the near future. With them, things will always be better in the near future – hence the term 'jam tomorrow' – and they operate on the basis that by the time the promised 'tomorrow' arrives either they will have moved on to a new post, or the circumstances in which they are working will have changed to such an extent that they will not be held to account for their original strategy. Watching the 'jam tomorrow' brigade operate is almost like being the spectator of some new sport or art form. They are masters at putting off the day on which they have to deliver, and in the meantime they create immense activity (project groups, working parties and implementation plans) that attract large groups of supporters who genuinely believe that they are involved in critically important work.

Then there are those whose approach to policy and strategy appears to be driven by a touch of megalomania and egomania. For them, strategy formulation resembles something close to world domination for their service, and their forecasts for performance can even enter the realm of make-believe. I have seen this approach in many major organisations, but two examples will suffice here. One of the examples is a large manufacturing conglomeration, and the other is an international institution involved in developing health policy. Their claims beggared belief – one was going to swamp the world with its product and the other was going to achieve a radical transformation in the lives of countless millions. They seemed to be oblivious to the 'weaknesses' and 'threats' (to take the 'W' and 'T' out of SWOT analysis) of their strategic plans, and regarded any counter-argument as pessimistic and negative thinking and not in keeping with the positive outlook associated with the *raison d'être* of their organisation. Anyone who attempted to point out that the Emperor did not have any clothes was immediately labelled 'not one of us' and risked becoming an organisational outcast. Needless to say, both strategies came to grief, but one of the organisations managed to explain it away, in a similar manner to the 'jam tomorrow' practitioner, by explaining that the environment in which they were operating had changed dramatically and they could not have anticipated those changes under any circumstances. The other organisation teetered on the edge of bankruptcy and is now mainly famous for the extent of its downsizing programme, rather than for its products.

CONCLUSION

Remember Nasrudin? He spent his time and effort looking for his key in places where there was more light, and where people could see his industry, but where his chances of succeeding in his mission were zero.

His story should serve as a parable for managers everywhere and a challenge to check whether new strategies, or departmental reorganisations, or the introduction of new approaches, are an act 'in the light' rather than one that addresses the fundamental issues that they are facing. They need to ask themselves, and to ask themselves honestly, where and how their organisation and its people lost their 'key'. This is the only way in which effective change can become a reality.

The problem often lies with the core beliefs and behaviours of their team. Every time I visit the USA I am impressed by their positive attitude to customer service. When I am in France, I am astonished by their veneration for food and wine and the entire eating experience. But have you been to Paris Disneyland and seen the reluctance with which they attempt to adopt the 'have a nice day' American-based culture of Disney? It should be a clear lesson to all of us – instructing a workforce to utter some well-chosen words is not the same as bringing about a fundamental cultural change. We accept that fact, yet there are managers who will act as if, with a little reorganisation, some superficially applied new concept, and the announcement of a new policy or strategy – hey presto, all will be well in my organisation . . . but probably next year or the year after.

There are times in healthcare organisations when the issues that need to be tackled concern fundamental core beliefs and behaviours, yet the ever-optimistic manager, driven by the need to be seen to be taking proactive action, decides to reorganise the department. This is a manager of action, but action that will most likely prove to be futile in a short while. The tragedy is that these managers – albeit a minority – genuinely believe that reordering some posts on an organisational chart will fundamentally change the behaviour of their people. How sad this is.

They are working in the light instead of looking in the house.

Key actions

1 Try not to fall into the trap of treating only the symptoms of a problem. It really is important to identify and deal with the underlying causes.
2 Please think long and hard about the parable of Nasrudin and then answer this question honestly: 'Do I ever look outside the house and, if so, why do I do it?'
3 Here is another question: 'When you introduce a new strategy or initiative do you see it through or are you a gatherer of "moose heads"?'

REFERENCES

1 Mintzberg H (1989) *Mintzberg on Management.* The Free Press, New York.
2 Senge PM (1990) *The Fifth Discipline: the art and practice of the learning organization.* Century Business, London.
3 Senge PM (1990) The leader's new work: building learning organizations. *Sloan Manag Rev.* 32(1): 7–22.
4 Townsend R (1971) *Up the Organisation.* Coronet, Philadelphia, PA.
5 Mintzberg H (1979) *The Structuring of Organisations.* Prentice Hall, Englewood Cliffs, NJ.
6 Handy C (1995) *Gods of Management: the changing work of organisations.* Arrow, London.
7 Morgan G (1998) *Images of Organisation: the executive edition.* Berrett-Koehler, San Francisco and Sage, Thousand Oaks, CA.
8 Welch J and Byrne JA (2001) *Jack.* Headline, London.
9 Gerstner LV (2002) *Who Says Elephants Can't Dance?* HarperCollins, London.
10 Morgan G (1993) *Imaginization: the art of creative management.* Sage, London.

CHAPTER 9

Personal growth: seven essential steps

Anathema is the best word I can think of to describe my reaction when I see books claiming to contain the 'three essential steps to success' or the 'four aspects of perfect management'. They make me want to issue a solemn denunciation concerning the legitimacy of such books. I made up the titles I quoted, at least I think I did, but books with similar titles and making similar claims occupy far too many management bookshelves. Management and its various components are far too complicated to condense into a 'five steps for this' or 'three steps for that' approach. How can it be possible to take an issue as complex as leadership, or the management of change, condense it into a number of simple steps and then try to convince busy healthcare managers that they can become an expert within 100 or so pages of text and a week or so of experience. Despite my feelings of condemnation for such titles, it seems that each week more and more books of this type are being displayed in stores claiming to be serious bookshops. What is even more depressing is that the top 10 sales of management texts, published in reputable journals, are most likely to contain quick-fix answer books – quick fixes to some of the thorniest problems of organisational life.

To make matters worse, I confess that I have bought some of these books myself. Sometimes the purchase has been made in a slightly superior manner, but there have been times when I have bought them for their simple yet possibly effective insights into difficult issues that might help a client. So you can imagine my embarrassment and sense of hypocrisy when I chose a title for this chapter on personal growth that included the phrase *seven essential steps*. My reason for choosing such a title was simple. As I wrote down my ideas on personal growth and went through various texts and personal experiences, it became perfectly obvious to me that the best way of communicating the various ideas was to cast them as the seven essential steps to personal growth. Even the word *growth* caused me some difficulty, as I could have used the word *development* – this is after all a chapter about personal development – but somehow the word *growth* seemed more appropriate, so I have risked sounding as if I am communicating through the genre of self-help books. I am also discomforted by the thought that, after reading this chapter, people will assimilate the seven steps and then be disappointed when their healthcare career does not blossom as quickly as they expected. So before I launch into the seven steps, one thing needs to be made absolutely clear. Although the seven points are robust, based on sound experience of applying them in many areas of the health service and a theoretical understanding of personal development, they are nevertheless seven steps that need to be practised not just for a month or two, but over one's entire career. They are seven steps for a lifetime.

The unease I experience with writers who promise spectacular transformations by following three or four principles does not include the work of Stephen Covey, even though one of his worldwide best-sellers is called *The Seven Habits of Highly Effective People*. Covey actually emphasises the point I have made and, despite the 'catchy' title of his book, his work is the very antithesis of the style I have been criticising. In the introduction to his book on leadership, Covey emphasises the importance of taking an in-depth systematic approach to the issue of development:

> I have long advocated a natural, gradual, day-by-day, step-by-step, sequential approach to personal development. My feeling is that any product or program – whether it deals with losing weight or mastering skills – that promises 'quick, free, instant and easy' results is probably not based on correct principles. Yet virtually all advertising uses one or more of these words to entice us to buy. Small wonder many of us are addicted to 'quick-fix' approaches to personal development.[1]

So here are the seven steps. They will last you a lifetime, you will need to practise them continually, and if you are ever tempted to believe that you have mastered them, it is likely that you have failed to understand the full extent of the steps you needed to take. They are some challenge, and I wish you well.

STEP 1: TAKE RESPONSIBILITY

This is the fundamental starting point, and it is a startling message – when it comes to your growth, *you* are the person who is ultimately responsible for it. This is an essential state of mind to possess, and without it you run the risk of becoming one of those people who constantly complains that their organisation or manager does nothing to develop them. That is whining and it is pitiful. I realise there are healthcare organisations where there is less commitment to developing staff than in others, but even in those organisations it is essential that individuals realise that they are the ones who are ultimately responsible for their own growth. You may think that I am being unrealistic and that it is impossible for a person to develop him- or herself in an organisation that will not send him or her on a course or pay the fees for a qualification. If that is what you think, then by the time you finish reading this chapter you will need to redefine your understanding of the words *development* and *growth*. When you have read this chapter you will understand that development and growth can take place in a multitude of different ways, and that even in an organisation that does not develop its people in a systematic way there are always opportunities to learn, develop and grow. And of course you always have the option of leaving your present healthcare organisation if it has a less than perfect record for development.

Have you noticed how a 'victim mentality' is creeping into so many parts of our society, with more and more people ducking their responsibility, moral or otherwise, and claiming that they acted in the way they did, or didn't act at all, because of certain external circumstances? It has become a perfectly legitimate everyday defence mechanism: 'I did it because of X or Y or Z.' It seems to be a reaction that is spreading into even more parts of society, and the victim mentality can also be found in organisations. The best antidote to the victim malaise is to be found in the world of occupational psychology. Occupational psychologists talk about the *locus of control*, and ask individuals to consider whether control over various factors in their lives exists outside their power to influence it, or within their power to exercise control over it. If it is within their power to influence it, then they ought to be able, or at least more able, to control it. In much the same way, helping people to see that much of what they blame others for is actually within their control is a fundamental step in personal growth and development.

At this stage you may not be convinced of this argument, but as you read the remainder of the chapter you should see the point itself being developed and, as a result, become committed to taking responsibility for your own growth. Are you in charge or do you feel like a victim? Are you in charge or do you sometimes say that your hospital or whatever does little to develop you? I know that there are poor organisations when it comes to development, but you can overcome them and see personal growth happen before your very own eyes. If the healthcare organisation that you work for is truly dreadful in terms of development, then you have the option of leaving it and finding a job elsewhere. Take control. You must be the person in charge.

STEP 2: ATTITUDES TO LEARNING

So you feel responsible for your own development. Good, then the next step will take you further on. This step concerns the right attitudes to learning.

One of the simplest yet most profound demonstrations of the way in which learning and management interact comes from the work of John Burgoyne.[2] He developed what is called the *MLml framework*, where 'M' denotes formal, explicit, deliberate management; 'L' denotes formal, explicit, deliberate learning; 'm' denotes informal management, and 'l' denotes informal learning.

In this model, Burgoyne distinguishes between 'formalised, institutionalised practices of management (M) and learning (L) and the equivalent practices in informal, naturally occurring management (m) and learning (l)'. 'M' refers to the formal activities of management in any organisation, such as formal positions, strategies or even committees, while 'm' refers to the everyday activities that take place in order to get things done in the organisation. 'L' refers to the formal courses or training events that are scheduled and where learning is clearly stated as an expected outcome, whereas 'l' refers to informal observations or practices that bring about learning.

Burgoyne takes his differentiation and starts to generate categories to show various dimensions of management and learning, and the principles he identifies can be applied to learning for people in all organisations. Some of his (numerous) categories are as follows:

➤ mM – informal, personal and private strategies that individuals and groups employ in order to deal with formal management systems
➤ Mm – formal management attempts to control informal management processes (e.g. attempts to manage culture)
➤ LL – formal research on and study of deliberate and explicit learning processes (e.g. in courses, etc.)
➤ lL – learning to cope with formal learning experiences and situations
➤ ll – informal understanding of informal learning processes.

These are merely a sample of the categories that can be generated and there are many more potential permutations that can be obtained by using, in combination, the letters ML, mL, lM or lm. The application of Burgoyne's point is really simple yet profound. In any organisation – and this is certainly true of healthcare organisations – there are examples of formal and informal management, and formal and informal learning, and there is an interplay between them. The challenge for the individual is to discover where these exist and to avail him- or herself of as many of the learning/management combinations as possible. When I first saw Burgoyne's work I was impressed, and I immediately saw the potential to demonstrate to delegates on NHS development programmes not only that personal growth is a personal responsibility, but also that it can be managed in various and flexible ways. So much development can come from the observation and analysis of informal management (m) and learning (l) and the interaction between them. The 'learner' may need a colleague or a mentor/ coach to help, but even without such support it is possible to reflect on what has been observed in an organisation. There are key learning questions to ask. Why was that aspect of management launched in a formal way and why did the other activity take place in an informal setting? Which approach was the more appropriate and what were the benefits of the respective methods? Why did those managers behave in that particular style and what would have happened if they had done things differently? Why does manager X seem more able to get things implemented than manager Y? How do successful managers go about having an informal word with someone rather than launching a full-blown strategic paper? The questions, and the learning, can go on and on. If there is an opportunity to discuss these issues with those who have been observed, this is an even better form of learning, as it is then possible to test assumptions and achieve quicker learning.

I encourage people to experiment with this framework – even to have fun with it – and to see how it helps learning and growth in both a practical and theoretical manner. It helps the 'learner' to discover why some managers are more successful than others; how they use personal and impersonal approaches; how they manage formally and manage informally, and when and why they do it. The amount of learning is boundless and, above all, it helps to show that informal learning is sometimes more appropriate than formal learning, and that no matter what limitations are placed on an individual within the healthcare organisation, they can still continue to learn and develop.

Action learning is a closely related concept. Around 1990, the participants in an NHS management development programme invited me to attend their end-of-course dinner. I readily accepted, as I had recently been appointed to a development role and wanted to demonstrate my commitment to them, even though it would mean a 200-mile drive for me from a speaking engagement at another conference. It would be a close call if I managed to arrive at their dinner on time. I managed it, with minutes to spare, and was ushered into the dining room and placed at the top table. I was tired, a little disorientated and, to my eternal shame, did not immediately appreciate that the octogenarian sitting next to me was none other than Reg Revans, the father of action learning and, in the field of learning, a man treated with something nigh on reverence. The conversation was entertaining, but I still wonder whether I made the most of what was a golden opportunity.

Revans is the man who pioneered the notion of action learning, and his book the *ABC of Action Learning*[3] is a classic. His belief that 'there can be no learning without action and no action without learning' is the stuff of folklore and, as Mike Pedlar, a man who has brought Revans' work to a wider audience, points out, 'he argues that observable behavioural change only take place when learners decide for themselves and when they have been faced with real issues'. Revans introduces us to the equation $L = P + Q$, where L denotes learning, P denotes the acquisition of programmed knowledge and Q denotes questioning insight. Pedlar, seeing a deeper meaning in Revans's formula, adds:

> Revans goes beyond the convention of teaching knowledge or 'P' as he symbolises it, and introduces what good philosophers and scientists have always done, that is to subject their knowledge of 'P' to fresh and tough questions or 'Q'. This way of penetrating one's understanding of something by introducing new questions removes the limitations of one's learning capacity and alleviates one's knowledge of one's own learning process.

This principle can be applied to all areas of work, and when introduced into a team setting it can be a powerful source of learning and growth. The returns on any effort put in are encouraging, and many a healthcare team has benefited beyond its expectations from the investment of first making action learning an agenda item at the end of their meetings, and secondly, arriving at a place where action learning becomes a natural habit and the way in which work is conducted in the department or indeed the whole organisation.

For many months after my dinner with Reg Revans we engaged in correspondence, and I remember well his spidery handwriting and the letters that started 'My Dear Prosser'. What surprised me about the correspondence was the sense that these letters were from a man who appeared disappointed that his work had not had a greater effect upon the workplace. In my replies I emphasised that he had had a major impact on the understanding of learning, and that his work had been a catalyst for that done by many others. I told him of ways in which his work was being applied within the health service, but I am not sure that I convinced him. It may be that his overall appreciation of his life's work was far more positive, or that I placed an undue emphasis on his comments, or it may be that he did not realise that the work of a prophet – for that is surely what he was – is not always fully accepted during his own lifetime. Revans deserves to be in the pantheon of learning greats.

From Revans to Garvin

David Garvin, the Harvard Business School writer, is another who recognises the true significance of learning. He writes:

> Teaching puts the instructor front and centre. Concepts and ideas flow from the top down or the centre out, and the focus is on knowledge transfer. Teachers are the experts . . . students are regarded as novices; their role is to absorb and accept. The effectiveness of the process is usually measured by the degree to which important information makes the trip from the first group to the second without distortion or loss . . . Knowledge is repackaged and repositioned, but *deeper learning is not achieved . . . A process designed to foster learning is quite different* [my italics] . . . New ways of thinking become the desired ends, not facts or frameworks. Discussion and debate replace ex-cathedra pronouncements . . . and success is measured by the degree to which students 'learn to learn'.[4]

'Learn to learn' is a critically important message, yet so many people fail to understand and apply this principle.

The third and final part of Step 2 concerns *mental habits*. This is based on the work of John Kotter,[5] another Harvard academic, and I have introduced it to great effect with groups of healthcare managers and clinicians in order to challenge their attitude to learning. Kotter describes what he calls mental habits that support lifelong learning. These consist of risk taking (a willingness to push oneself out of one's comfort zones), humble self-reflection (an honest assessment of one's successes and failures), solicitation of opinions (the aggressive collection of information and ideas from others), careful listening (the propensity to listen to others) and an openness to new ideas (the willingness to view life with an open mind).

These five points, which I have abbreviated, appear to be little more than common sense, but in my experience of using them extensively with managers and clinicians, they are profound when considered sincerely. They ask searching questions about the very nature of the way we work and learn. Sadly, there are too many people who are not prepared to engage in any activity, or any new way of tackling a problem, if there is any risk associated with it. Humility is not always to be found in vast quantities, and there is an alarming tendency to sweep failures under the corporate carpet and to pretend that they never took place. Asking the opinion of those who are likely to agree with one's own position is one thing, but true learning can often come from those who have a very different view from the one you happen to hold. Listening differs from hearing in that it involves an active component, a component that is usually effective when it is linked to reflection and action. And new ideas are a wonderful source of learning, and the fact that 80% of the ideas might be 'off the wall' should not

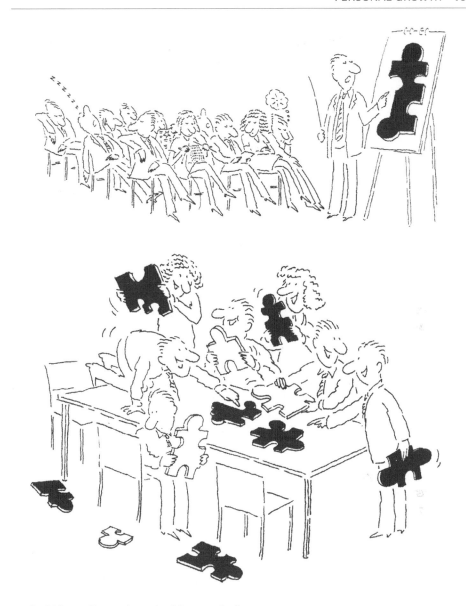

© Jüri Kann. Reproduced with permission.

prevent a healthcare organisation from actively promoting the notion of ideas and seeing such practice as a sign of a fertile and imaginative organisational environment.

STEP 3: KNOW YOURSELF

Karl Wallenda, the great tightrope aerialist, once said, 'The only time I feel truly alive is when I walk the tightrope . . .' Shortly after Wallenda fell to his death in 1978 (traversing a 75-foot-high tightrope in downtown San Juan, Puerto Rico), his wife, also an aerialist, discussed the fateful San Juan walk, 'perhaps his most dangerous.' She recalled, 'All Karl thought about for three straight months prior to it was falling. It was the first time he'd ever thought about that, and it seemed to me that he put all his energy into not falling, not into walking the tightrope.' Mrs Wallenda went on to say that her husband even went so far as to personally supervise the installation of the tightrope, making certain that the guy-wires were secure, 'something he had never even thought of before.'[6]

The first time I read the story of Karl Wallenda it had a profound effect on me. It was one of the moments when you know that you have been spoken to in a way that reaches deep inside you. I had never heard of Wallenda before this, and so it seems insincere if I attempt to offer any sense of condolence for what happened to him. Wallenda's story speaks clearly about two issues of personal growth.

The first is that there are some activities which we undertake in our lives – whether as a part of our work, or with our family, or through our involvement in the community – that make us feel *truly alive* (to use Wallenda's phrase). In terms of work these may be rare moments for most people, but for some, the fortunate ones, these moments are experienced frequently. Recognising what these activities are is an integral part of *knowing yourself* and doing your best to place yourself in a job that meets these needs and makes you feel truly alive. This may sound idealistic and out of touch with the realities of everyday life, but most of us have the opportunity to work in areas that involve an interaction with people, if that is what makes us feel *truly alive*, or to work as an accountant if we relish the prospect of dealing with figures all day, or in the community, or in the open air, or behind the wheel of an ambulance. Some people do not have this blessing, of course, but for most people there is an opportunity to get close to that ideal state even if it has to be found outside the workplace. Knowing yourself and placing yourself in a suitable job will help you to grow and develop into the person you ought to be – the person you have the potential to become.

The second lesson to draw from this story is the danger of concentrating on the detail, even the minutiae, of the job and failing to concentrate your resources and time on the big picture – which is usually the very reason for the job's existence. This is the best way to impress your bosses, through the medium of excellent performance. I have sympathy for Mr Wallenda, and I know that if I was ever crazy enough to try and walk a tightrope I would want to check every single centimetre of the rope and all of the attachments. I would never agree to walk a rope because I know I would be mesmerised by the prospect of what could go wrong. This is probably the same reason that I have never attempted to become an entrepreneur – because of the overwhelming prospect of what could go wrong – and why successful entrepreneurs appear to be able to concentrate on the big picture, rather than the minutiae of the job. It is an important part of knowing yourself.

The story of Karl Wallenda teaches two very crucial points in terms of knowing yourself. What work should you undertake to make you feel *truly alive*? And what should you do in order to keep seeing the big picture and remain in a positive state of mind?

Ways to discover yourself

There are safer ways than tightrope walking to discover these principles, to help you to discover what is likely to make you feel *truly alive*. In my experience the following tests, appraisals and assessment methods have a particular utility, and although I have an attachment to these four well-known techniques, my real purpose in describing them is to encourage you to investigate ways in which you can find out more about yourself, and turn that invaluable knowledge into a career that is truly fulfilling.

The Myers-Briggs Type Indicator[7]

The Myers-Briggs Type Indicator (MBTI), developed by Katharine C Briggs and Isabel Briggs Myers, is based on a personality framework that helps people to explore their preferences for taking in information and making decisions. The framework also looks at where people prefer to focus their attention and how they prefer to live their life. It gives information about the preferred style of working and interacting with other people. There are no right or wrong answers, and all personality profiles are equally valid and the feedback concentrates on likely strengths and positive qualities, and as such is always seen to be constructive. When I became an academic I no longer had the luxury of relying on my team of NHS occupational psychologists, so I decided to train in MBTI. I qualified and found it a deeply rewarding process, as it gave me a greater insight into myself and other people. For years I had been aware of the basic model, but now I understand far more about the source of energy for introverts and extroverts (E and I), how people take in information (S and N), make decisions (T and F) and relate to their environment (J and P). Many more things make sense.

The FIRO-B

The FIRO-B (Fundamental Interpersonal Relationship Orientation – Behaviour) instrument[8] provides another useful revelation of how people behave. First developed in the 1950s by Will Schutz as a part of his research for the US Navy, it is based on the theory that beyond our needs for survival, food, shelter and warmth we have distinct interpersonal needs that make us feel comfortable. Although we are not necessarily bound by typical behaviours, being aware of natural tendencies allows us to choose whether a particular behaviour is or is not appropriate at a specific time. The three dimensions of the FIRO-B (which need to remain undisclosed, as prior knowledge of the dimensions may damage the benefit of the questionnaire) are then applied to the way in which we express ourselves and the way in which we want others to behave towards us. This provides a fascinating insight and is only one of the FIRO suite of diagnostic instruments, as many more recent options are now available.

The Johari window

For years I treated the Johari window concept (*see* Figure 9.1) with a degree of scorn. I have always been sceptical of diagnostic devices presented as a four-box solution to complex problems. As far as I was concerned, the underlying ideas in the Johari window were far too simple. However, as I extended my list of health

Unknown to others	Known to others	
Known to self, unknown to others	Known to self and others	Known to self
Unknown to self or others	Unknown to self, known to others	Unknown to self

FIGURE 9.1 The Johari window

service and public-sector coaching clients, and developed my understanding of personality type, the Johari window began to grow on me.

During a coaching session with a manager, clinician or civil servant, it provided a meaningful hook on which to hang many relevant points of feedback. Its utility increased further when it was used to illustrate the impact of self-awareness and an awareness of others during formal and informal communication. If you imagine two Johari windows side by side, and consider them to denote two people communicating with each other, then it is relatively easy to imagine how communication can go awry – person A's 'known to self, unknown to others' communicates to person B's 'unknown to self, known to others' and person B's 'known to self, known to others' communicates to person A's 'unknown to self, unknown to others'. Communication pandemonium can break out.

Such a diagnostic aid can be used to full effect when asking a client to consider how they are viewed by those receiving their communication, and the impact that this impression has on the effectiveness of their communication and the initiative they are trying to introduce. Most clinicians and managers find it extremely helpful, and it should play a full part in the quest to know yourself.

360-degree appraisal

The final example is 360-degree appraisal, and here I rely entirely on the experiences of clients, who have found it to be a worthwhile experience. There are many proprietary applications of the basic idea, some good and others a little suspect, and 360-degree appraisal provides the opportunity to discover, fairly painlessly, what your boss, colleagues and those who work for you think of your managerial style and performance. There are limitations to the process, including the degree of honesty used by those who work with you (and especially by those who work for you), but even allowing for those limitations there is much to be gained from this approach.

STEP 4: LEARNING, DIAGNOSIS AND PRESCRIPTION

The fourth step is to understand something about your learning styles and preferences. Most people understand that there are very different learning styles, based on their experience of life and education. From our schooldays we understand that there are some people who can leave their studying until a short while before the examinations and then astound everyone by their ability to cram vast amounts of knowledge into their brains in a matter of a few days. They also possess the ability to regurgitate this knowledge for the benefit of the examiner, but whether they remember those facts a few weeks later is questionable. For others the annual examination became a time of nightmares. They learned about things in a very different way. For them, the way they learned was associated more with steady work over a period of time, or relating theory to practice and applying it in a particular way, rather than with 'cramming' one or two days before an examination. This is one of the reasons that so many people of my generation were considered failures in their secondary education and only blossomed when they left formal and set-in-their-ways educational environments. I well remember the research director of a major UK company telling me that he had more PhDs than 'O'-levels! He had been a victim of the 'only one way to learn' regime that dominated his generation. Thankfully, schools are now far better at recognising different approaches to learning, and often provide students with a greater variety of learning experiences and assess them in more appropriate ways. Despite this enlightened approach, I remain of the view that the terror of examinations is still far too prevalent.

To discover a respectable theory underlying the ways in which people learn is a relief to many individuals. I am aware of the literature underpinning the behaviourist, cognitive, humanist and constructivist theories,[9] but wish to narrow my examples to those regarded as having practical utility by managers and clinicians themselves. Whether you are a disciple of Kolb and his classification of learners as having a preference for concrete experience, active conceptualisation, active experimentation or reflective observation; or of Honey and Mumford's classification of activists, reflectors, pragmatists and theorists; or of Felder-Silverman's five classifications of sensing or intuitive learners, visual or verbal learners, inductive or deductive learners, active or reflective learners, and sequential or global learners; or of the Herrman brain-dominance instrument that classifies learners' thinking into four different modes (logical thinkers, sequential thinkers, emotional thinkers and holistic thinkers)[10] it is such a comfort – and a valuable insight – to discover that there is a learning style to suit each person.

Step 4: Part I

Therefore the first part of Step 4 is to discover the most appropriate learning style for you, and then to design a development experience to match it. Despite this basic fact it is astonishing to witness the number of programmes, at highly regarded establishments, that remain wedded to one particular style of learning. In the mid-1990s I attended an international healthcare executive programme at a leading US university, and the entire formal learning experience consisted of wall-to-wall lectures from faculty and visiting dignitaries. There seemed to be a lack of awareness both of the notion of learning styles and of the learning that could take place between the programme delegates if more time had been allowed for it. Development programmes need to recognise that activists will 'thrive on the challenge of new experiences', reflectors will 'like to consider all possible angles and implications before making a move', theorists will be 'keen on basic assumptions, principles, theories, models and system thinking', and pragmatists will 'positively search out new ideas or techniques which might apply in their situation'.[11] Fortunately, there are more and more programmes, or other development options, that recognise this important principle.

Step 4: Part 2

By and large, managers tend to be people of action – they want to change things, to make things happen, and they often find it difficult to spend time thinking about the way things are done in their organisation. Walk into any manager's office and it is unusual to find many books on their shelves, unless there is some management best-seller that they bought on a business trip and haven't quite finished reading yet. What so many managers find difficult is to programme into their diaries a time for reflection. This is not really a surprising fact if most of the managers were appointed for their track record of being an activist/pragmatist man or woman of action.

Yet reflection is a key activity. Clutterbuck and Megginson[12] developed the concept of personal reflective space (PRS), which they define as 'the seized opportunity to develop personal insight through uninterrupted and purposeful reflective activity', and their six-step process helps executives and managers to practise the art of reflective practice. Burgoyne[13] shows that 'where practitioners can render some plausible account of how they perform – in other words, articulate a theory of their practice, they become *reflective practitioners* producing *reflective practice*'. He continues his argument by suggesting that 'among the advantages of being a reflective practitioner is the ability to transfer skills . . . to others, and the possibility of working out how to adapt the theory and practice to a changed circumstance rather than relying on intuition and trial and error'.

Some people need a formal process, a step-by-step guide, to help with reflection, but for others it seems to be a natural ability and they prefer a less structured approach, and some managers practise reflection when walking, driving or having a bath! The tragedy consists of those managers who find little benefit in reflecting on how they and their organisation are performing. They are unable, or so it seems, to ask fundamentally important questions such as the following. What can I/we learn from a particular achievement? What can I/we learn from something that went wrong? How did I/we handle a tricky issue? Could I/we have done it better or differently, and what outcomes would that alternative action have produced? The response, far too often, is anything but reflection. A man or woman of action does not have the time for such mundane activities, or so it seems – they need the constant 'rush' of pressing on to the next action free of any doubt in their innate ability to make things happen.

Step 4: Part 3

The growth in executive coaching and mentoring is the glorious exception to lamenting the absence of reflection in management practice. Pedants and semanticists prefer a clear differentiation between the terms *coach* and *mentor*, but I use the terms interchangeably, as the best coaches and mentors use a variety of techniques and refuse to get hung up on the niceties of a particular title. A range of literature has been published showing the benefits of coaches and mentors and illustrating the main principles behind the concepts. Much of it resonates with the work of Clutterbuck and Megginson,[14] and their views on the common roles of a mentor as being a sounding board (giving honest feedback on how the manager plans to tackle an issue), a critical friend (someone who is willing and able to say openly those things that colleagues are reluctant to say), a listener (someone who can offer encouragement and a listening ear), a counsellor (an empathetic listener, with the reflective and questioning skills necessary to help the executive to analyse problems and opportunities), a career adviser (helping the executive to think through career and development options), a networker (providing the executive with access to helpful networks and individual contacts) and a coach (helping the executive to make personal change happen, especially at the behavioural level).

The concept of mentor capitalists is also growing in popularity. Leonard and Swap[15] show how these mentor capitalists help unseasoned, first-time entrepreneurs to create and refine a business model, find top talent, build business processes, test their ideas in the marketplace and attract funding. Although all mentor capitalists refuse to make decisions on behalf of the entrepreneurs, the teaching (an interesting use of the word 'teaching' in a US journal to explain mentoring) methods of the mentors vary substantially. They include learning by doing, Socratic learning (a series of challenging questions and responses), stories with a moral (based on the mentor's experience of personal maxims), rules of thumb (experiential business principles), specific directives (in support of an executive decision) and learning by observing. It is a fascinating development that could be adapted to the healthcare world and bring much benefit.

Research from the Industrial Society,[16] an organisation now rebranded as the Work Foundation, shows that the areas where coaching can be of most value are the development of knowledge management, during mergers, in times of cultural change, and in relation to issues of work-life balance. The same article wisely states that for coaching to be effective, the 'coachee' (a ghastly word!) has to be receptive, adaptable, open, disciplined and non-confrontational. These terms are self-explanatory and they square with people's experience of coaching in many walks of life and at various levels of seniority.

Step 4: Part 4

This is the final part of Step 4. Over the years, I have advised hundreds of healthcare staff about their personal development. One of the things that never ceases to surprise me is the number of times the conversation starts with the person saying 'I need to do an MBA', or 'I think I should go on a management course at Ashridge or Henley (or somewhere similar)', or 'I need to change my job'. What becomes clear after a short period of discussion is that the reasoning they have used to reach their conclusion is suspect, and in some cases there is little evidence of any systematic thinking at all. In other words, they have fallen into the common trap of putting prescription before diagnosis – they have decided through some incoherent process the answer to an undefined question! Imagine visiting a doctor who advises you to take a particular medication without asking any questions before issuing the prescription. The same principle holds true for development – it is essential to thoroughly diagnose the development needs before jumping to some conclusion as to what the answer (the prescription) might be. The process of diagnosing the development needs is not rocket technology, but it is a fundamental step if there is to be any hope of engaging in development that is appropriate for both the individual and the healthcare organisation.

The starting point in this process is to ask yourself and others in the organisation – including your boss, if the relationship is one in which learning and development are valued – what the principal requirements of the job are. This should not become an attempt to draw up a list of managerial competencies in a mechanical way, but it should form the basis for an honest discussion of what is required to perform the job well. Then you should take a long hard look at yourself, hopefully with the co-operation of your boss and your colleagues once more, and this might even be an opportunity for meaningful use of the 360-degree appraisal process. You might be fortunate enough to have access to someone who is an expert in management and personal and organisation development. What you will discover is that there are only eight or nine different development activities available (examples include, in no particular order, formal education or management courses; coaching/mentoring; secondment; a project; shadowing a senior figure; action learning in some form or other, and other variations on the theme). The skill of the management development/ organisation development expert will lie in agreeing with you the best option(s) to suit your needs, personal circumstances, learning style and personality. From there on it should be plain sailing.

STEP 5: THE POWER OF NEW EXPERIENCES

To illustrate this step I want to relate three stories – two from real-life experiences and one from the world of theatre.

STORY 9.1[17]

My youngest son Simon won a goldfish at the local fair and brought it home. Sam the goldfish was a real tiddler, but far too big for the jar he was in. So we put him in a goldfish bowl we had stored in the garage for many years. Each day he was fed, and sometimes he was fed twice or even three times a day. After a few weeks he had grown far too big for the bowl, so we put him in a small aquarium that had been given to us by our neighbour. He was fed regularly, his water was oxygenated with some suitable vegetation, and he became quite a lovable character. On a couple of occasions he became so excited when we came home that he managed to jump out of the water and land on the kitchen floor. Sam continued to grow, and we bought him a large aquarium. As my son got older he became somewhat bored with Sam, and we became increasingly concerned about the lack of space Sam had to swim in. So we gave him to a neighbour who had a garden pond. Sam loved it, continued to grow and ended up the size of a small trout. For Sam the goldfish there was also an unexpected benefit. We had always thought that he was a 'boy' goldfish, although I can't quite understand how we came to that conclusion, so you can imagine our surprise on a visit to Sam to discover that *she* had given birth. Immediately Sam became Samantha.

Personal development is based on the same principle. Not surprisingly I call it the 'Sam the goldfish principle', and I've seen it happen time and time again to people. You place someone in a larger environment, where they are 'fed' and supported in a sensible way, and before your very eyes they start to grow – not physically, but in terms of influence, contribution and impact. When the time is right they need to be placed in an even larger environment. As with Sam, this is done for their benefit, but unlike Sam, it benefits others and only happens with their agreement. I have seen this happen in all walks of life – nurses, doctors, managers and many others – and I never cease to be amazed by the potential within people to grow, and the fact that this potential is so often untapped by them and those charged with looking after them.

STORY 9.2

J Sterling Livingston developed a magnificent metaphor for personal growth when he borrowed from the experiences of Eliza Doolittle in George Bernard Shaw's *Pygmalion* (or *My Fair Lady*, if you saw the film version) to write an article on personal development.[18] Towards the end of the film there is a poignant scene in which Eliza, following her triumph in transforming herself from a Cockney flower girl into a member of elevated society, speaks about the way she is treated by Colonel Pickering and Professor Higgins:

> You see, really and truly, apart from the things anyone can pick up (the dressing and the proper way of speaking, and so on) the difference between a lady and a flower girl is not how she behaves but how she's treated. I shall always be a flower girl to Professor Higgins because he always treats me as a flower girl and always will, but I know I can be a lady to you because you always treat me as a lady and always will.

This is a moving scene, and so typical of how many people are treated even in healthcare organisations when they have stayed there 'man and boy', to use a trusted archaism. It is very hard to be in an organisation such as a hospital as a senior person, or as someone capable of achieving high rank, when there are those in the organisation, even if they are in lower grades, who remember you as the green, wet-behind-the-ears and probably slightly arrogant youngster who thought he had the answer for everything. There are notable exceptions to this rule, of course, and there are inspiring stories of those who started on the shop-floor and worked their way up to run the organisation. But the general rule seems to be that if you want to be treated in accordance with the status you now deserve, you do seem to have to move to another organisation or, at the very least, to another part of the same healthcare organisation.

I once told this story about Eliza at a workshop where I was speaking to a group of clinicians and allied health professionals. As I came to the end of the tale I noticed that one of the delegates had tears in her eyes, and she told us a moving story. In addition to her 'day job' she was a dedicated amateur dramatics performer, and only a few months earlier had played the part of Eliza Doolittle in a performance of *My Fair Lady* at a local theatre. She knew the script so well that she was still able to repeat sections of it, to the joy of all the people at the workshop. However, what had brought tears to her eyes was the fact that she had never applied the principle to her own career. As soon as I had started to use the metaphor it became crystal clear to her that her boss saw her far more as a 'flower girl' than as an 'educated and cultured lady'. For her it was a turning point, and it became a motivation to do something about her career. I never came into contact with her again, but I really hope that she is now being treated in a way that respects her talents and potential contribution.

The first story concerned how an individual can grow in the right environment, and the second story concerned how the growth of an individual can be stunted by someone else's perception of him or her. The third story concerns the growth we can experience when we decide not to limit ourselves to preconceived and often ill-founded preconceptions about what represents reality.

STORY 9.3

> Harry (not his real name) is a good friend and former work colleague of mine, and about four times a year we have lunch together. On one of these occasions as we were walking to the restaurant, on a cold and wet day, Harry noticed two 2p coins lying on the pavement. As he spied them he bent down, picked them up, placed them in his pocket and said in his educated Scottish brogue 'I can't stand things going to waste'. I didn't show my surprise at the eager way in which he pocketed the two 2p coins. We went into the restaurant and spent an enjoyable hour or so together and, as it was his turn to pay, he called for the bill, paid in cash and gave the waitress a £3 tip, which represented about 15% of the bill.

When I tell this story to groups of people I usually pause momentarily after the words '. . . educated Scottish brogue . . .', and invariably it produces some laughter as people immediately jump to what they consider to be the obvious conclusion – yet further evidence that Scottish people are careful with their money (to use a well-known euphemism). I have never told this story in Scotland, but I know that when it comes to Harry, and probably the vast majority of Scottish people, such accusations of thriftiness could not be further from the truth. I know from years of experience that Harry is an extremely generous person and that his action with the two 2p coins was nothing more than what he said it was – he didn't want to see things being wasted.

The story is instructive because it reminds us that it is all too easy to jump to conclusions, especially when they are based on stereotypical (and in extreme cases, even racist or sexist) prejudices. We all know the attributes that are sometimes ascribed to certain nationalities, or professions, or particular types of people, and apart from their discriminatory nature, they also rob us of the benefits of seeing people for what they really are, rather than seeing them from some prejudicial viewpoint.

The ladder of inference

Appreciating and then applying the concepts contained within Argyris's *ladder of inference*[19] (*see* Figure 9.2) is an important step in overcoming any potential bias and experiencing the benefit of new insights.

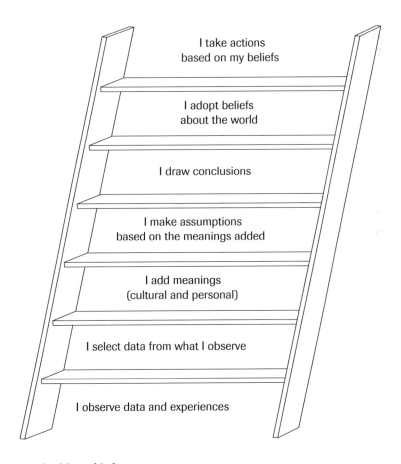

FIGURE 9.2 Ladder of inference
Source: Argyris C (1993) *Knowledge for Action. A guide to overcoming organizational barriers.* Jossey-Bass, San Francisco, CA, and John Wiley and Sons, New York.

Argyris describes the ladder of inference as:

> a hypothetical model of how individuals make inferences. They begin by experiencing some relatively observable data, such as conversation. This is rung 1 of the ladder. They make inferences about the meanings embedded in the words (rung 2). They often do this in milliseconds, regardless of whether they agree with the meanings. Then they impose their meanings on the actions they believe the other person intends (rung 3). For example, they attribute reasons or causes for the actions. They may also evaluate the actions as effective or ineffective. Finally, the attributions or evaluations they make are consistent with their theory-in-use about effective action (rung 4).

The idea of the ladder of inference has been applied in many settings, and has over time, as Figure 9.2 illustrates, attracted an additional two rungs. As Ross[20] shows, the ladder challenges a world of self-generating beliefs that remain largely untested. As a result, our ability to achieve what we really want is diminished by our feelings that:
➤ our beliefs are the truth
➤ the truth is obvious
➤ our beliefs are based on real data
➤ the data that we select are the real data.

This is what happens to people when I tell them the story of my Scottish friend Harry. They jump to conclusions and so miss the real truth and the benefit of seeing what a generous person Harry actually is. They miss out on so much, and these hasty conclusions are evident throughout the world of work, and as such cause people to miss out on many new experiences. Being aware of the dangers lurking within the ladder of inference allows us to act differently and, again as Ross shows us, to improve communication through reflection in three ways:
➤ by becoming more aware of our own thinking and reasoning (reflection)
➤ by making our thinking and reasoning more visible to others (advocacy)
➤ by inquiring into others' thinking and reasoning (inquiry).

The ladder of inference is used mainly as a tool to facilitate organisational learning, but it can also be used in the context of personal growth. As we learn not to jump to conclusions about the motives of people, we ensure that we are able to learn better from new experiences and from new insights that we had not seen before.

STEP 6: THE TRIANGLE OF PERFORMANCE

It was an *eureka* moment. I was browsing through a book on management consultancy by someone with the slightly exotic name of Calvert Markham,[21] and he was describing the '. . . three factors that combine to influence the selling performance of a professional: . . . technical skills, interpersonal skills and selling skills'. He had drawn a triangle in the text with each of the three factors as one side of the triangle, and the words *selling performance* in the centre of the triangle. I was not that interested, but then I read these words:

> The area of the triangle depends on the length of all three sides, so if the length of one side is nil, then the area will be nil. If the area of the triangle represents sales performance, all three skills must be represented to achieve a satisfactory standard of sales performance.

That was the *eureka* moment, and I saw immediately that what he had claimed for sales performance was also true for personal development. People with three dimensions to their job (and I shall show later that most people do have three dimensions to their job) must pay attention to all three factors if they want to grow. I saw that the area of the triangle represented overall personal development, and suddenly it became obvious that as one lengthens the size of an individual line, the overall area of the triangle increases. Similarly, if one of the sides of the triangle is neglected then the area of the triangle – one's overall personal effectiveness and growth – is restricted. If you remember your school mathematics classes then you will recall that to find the area of a triangle you needed to multiply half the length of the base by the perpendicular height of the triangle (do you remember $\frac{1}{2}b \times h$?). In personal growth terms you need to remember that every time you lengthen one of the sides of your triangle, the overall area, representing your personal growth, is increased. It was such an obvious point and yet such a revelation. My son, who is a mathematician, is impressed by the analogy but concerned by some of my mathematical imprecision.

What are the three factors that most people have as components of their work? If I use myself as an example, it is the ability to show that I can function as an academic, remain credible as a public-sector manager, and continue to operate close to the world of civil servants. In order to achieve this, I have worked hard to develop the skill of speaking the equivalent of three languages and sounding to the appropriate audience like an academic, a public-sector manager or a civil servant. For some people the three factors could be professional skill, business acumen and interpersonal relationships. For others they could be clinical or technical knowledge, an ability to show that what they do is relevant to the 'bottom line' of the organisation, and membership of a key team. For yet others the factors might be a specialist expertise, patient or client care, and the ability to relate their activities to the wider objectives of the healthcare organisation. There are many more examples, and I accept that there are some people who have four or even five factors that they have to manage in order to be seen to be effective. They might have to learn the equations for being a rectangle or a pentagon!

Markham makes another telling point. If the length of one side is nil, then the area will be nil. That explains why there are people in all healthcare organisations who are talented in many aspects of their job and yet who do not receive the advancement that they believe their talent merits. They may be well qualified professionally and possess many other fine personal qualities, but their understanding of the organisation and its needs is lamentable. Or they are first-rate team players, with a deep commitment to the organisation and its results, but there is some concern about whether their professional ability would pass muster against external competition. In other words, there is some concern about whether all three sides of their triangle are sufficiently developed.

The message could not be clearer. There is a need to discover the three sides of your work triangle (or perhaps even the four sides of your square) and to make sure that all of the sides are receiving treatment. You do not want to be a lopsided person – you need to be an equilateral triangle.

STEP 7: BEWARE

If you have taken responsibility for your own development, checked out your attitude to learning, taken steps to 'know yourself', gone through some diagnostic work, considered new experiences and reviewed your all-round performance, then there is a clear message for you – what works, works.

Beware of the so-called development expert who suggests to you that unless you are following a particular development pathway there is little hope for the career that you want to pursue. There may be times when it is expedient to attend a particular in-house development event, even if it is only for the networking opportunities, but you know far more than the average development expert about what will work for you. You have taken the time and effort to consider your development carefully from a number of perspectives, and you should be in a position to understand what works best for you.

Beware of those individuals who use the words *learning, training, knowledge* and *education* interchangeably as if they were one and the same thing. They are not. The need to take care in this area is exemplified by the work of two British academics, Cunningham and Davies,[22] who argue that:

> It is clear that . . . most of what managers learn about managing does not come from [structured courses or] programmes. They learn most from their day-to-day work, from colleagues, from observing other managers, and from sundry life experiences (e.g. travel). Nonetheless, questions of how to help managers learn more – and more effectively – tend to be focused on organised programmes.

They go on to show that there is an 'assumption that what is taught equals what is learned . . . and that the premise is that knowledge and skill transfer is relatively unproblematic'. They also show that for real learning to take place there is a need to provide individuals with opportunities to practise, to experience active engagement with their peer group, to have the chance to fail without punishment, and much else.

Mayo and Lank,[23] in a down-to-earth way, show that 'education is the exposure to new knowledge, concepts and ideas in a relatively programmed way', whilst 'learning is "student-need-centred" and starts with the beneficiary' and 'training . . . involves being shown a way of doing things'.

We all know that skills training is relatively easy. This morning I may have been unable to use spreadsheets on my computer, but as a result of a day's training I feel that I have mastered the technique. We also know that knowledge acquisition can take longer, but the process involved in acquiring the knowledge is tried and tested, and these days includes new techniques associated with e-learning. The difficult area to assess is whether real learning has taken place – learning that can change attitudes and behaviour. In this paragraph it is not my intention to enter a debate on the various issues surrounding learning. I am merely setting out to suggest that people should beware of any person who uses the terms *training*, *education* and *learning* interchangeably without any sense of understanding the very important differences between them.

Beware of individuals who try to advise on development when it is clear that they have not appreciated fully that the world of work has changed, and is continuing to change, almost beyond recognition. I realise that this is not the case everywhere, and that there are some areas where the old verities remain true, but even they will change one day. It is just that they are lagging behind the changes which are taking place in most healthcare organisations.

When I was in school the careers advisory service seemed somewhat inadequate, even in those days. Now it would seem ludicrous to suggest to a young person that they should join a high-street bank if they wanted to be guaranteed a job for life. Or to suggest that they should join a business with an eye to its excellent pension scheme – the idea would be laughed out of court. Or to think that young people, the so-called generation X, and the even younger generation Y, see life in the same way as the baby-boomers born after World War Two – this would show a remarkable lack of insight into how times have changed.

Thomas A Stewart, in his excellent book on intellectual capital,[24] identifies the impact on careers of the growth in the concept of intellectual capital within organisations. He demonstrates 'how much more ambiguous, now, are the paths ahead, and more various the strategies we might pursue' and he goes on to show how the new 'way of working affects career choices in six important ways'. The six ways he identifies (and they are fairly self-explanatory within the aims of this chapter) can be summarised as follows. A career is a series of gigs, not a series of steps. Project management is the furnace in which successful careers are forged. In the new organisation, power flows from expertise, not from position. Most roles in an organisation can be performed by either insiders or outsiders. Careers are made in markets (he means that you should think of yourself as a self-employed person even if you are a permanent member of staff) not in hierarchies. And the fundamental career choice is not between one healthcare organisation and another, but between specialising and generalising.

The final clear message is that you should beware of those who do not realise that the world of work has changed and that it is continuing to go through a revolution.

Key actions

1 There really is only one action, but the action can be considered as seven essential steps. If you are genuinely concerned about developing your healthcare career then you need to examine each of these seven steps and apply them to yourself. It would help if you had an adviser or colleague to help you with this.

REFERENCES

1 Covey SR (1991) *Principle-Centred Leadership*. Simon and Schuster, London.
2 Burgoyne J (1997) Introduction. In: J Burgoyne and M Reynolds (eds) *Management Learning: integrating perspectives in theory and practice*. Sage, London.
3 Revans R (1998) *ABC of Action Learning*. (The Mike Pedler Library). Lemos and Crane, London.
4 Garvin DA (2003) *Learning in Action*. Harvard Business School Press, Boston, MA.
5 Kotter J (1996) *Leading Change*. Harvard Business School Press, Boston, MA.
6 Bennis W (1994) *An Invented Life: reflections on leadership and change*. Perseus, Cambridge, MA.
7 'Myers-Briggs Type Indicator' and 'MBTI' are registered trademarks of the Myers-Briggs Type Indicator Trust. OPP Limited is licensed to use the trademarks in Europe.
8 FIRO-B is a trademark of CPP Inc., and OPP Limited is licensed to use the trademark in Europe.
9 Jones N (2004) *From Here to E-ternity: a learning journey*. Professorial Inaugural Lecture, University of Glamorgan, March 2004.
10 Schramm J (2002) *How Do People Learn?* Chartered Institute of Personnel and Development, London.
11 Mumford A and Gold J (2004) *Management Development: strategies for action*. Chartered Institute of Personnel and Development, London.
12 Clutterbuck D and Megginson D (1998) *Mentoring Executives and Directors*. Butterworth-Heinemann, Oxford.
13 Burgoyne J and Reynolds M (eds) (1997) *Management Learning: integrating perspectives in theory and practice*. Sage, London.
14 Clutterbuck D and Megginson D (1998) *Mentoring Executives and Directors*. Butterworth-Heinemann, Oxford.
15 Leonard D and Swap W (2000) Gurus in the garage. *Harvard Business Review*. November–December: 71–82.
16 Reported in *Bulletpoint*, July/August 2001; www.bulletpoint.com
17 Prosser S (2002) Personal development. *Prof Nurse*. 18: 117.
18 Livingston JS (1988) Pygmalion in management. *Harvard Business Review on Managing People*. Harvard Business School Press, Boston, MA.
19 Argyris C (1993) *Knowledge for Action. A guide to overcoming organizational barriers*. Jossey-Bass, San Francisco, CA, and John Wiley and Sons, New York. I have credited the source document, but the concept of the ladder of inference is available from many sources.
20 Ross R (1994) The ladder of inference. In: Senge, P., *et al.*, *The Fifth Discipline Fieldbook*. Nicholas Brealey, London.
21 Markham C (2001) *The Top Consultant*. Kogan Page, London.
22 Cunningham I and Davies G (1997) Problematic premises, presumptions, presuppositions and practices in management education and training. In: J Burgoyne and M Reynolds (eds) *Management Learning: integrating perspectives in theory and practice*. Sage, London.
23 Mayo A and Lank E (1994) *The Power of Learning*. Chartered Institute of Personnel and Development, London.
24 Stewart TA (1998) *Intellectual Capital*. Nicholas Brealey, London.

CHAPTER 10

Actions speak louder than words

When all is said and done, often more is said than done.

Anonymous

Words can have a dramatic effect on individuals, on groups of people and even on a nation. They can be a source of inspiration, driving people on to feats they once thought impossible; they can be a powerful force for good, bringing about dramatic change in the fortunes of a country; and, as we have seen in the tragic history of many totalitarian regimes, they can be misused and become a means of evil intent and purpose.

Among Winston Churchill's innumerable achievements is the fact that he was recognised to be an orator with few equals. Can you imagine the scene in June 1940 when he stood up in the House of Commons, during some of the darkest days of World War Two for the British people, and uttered the following memorable words?

> We shall not flag or fail. We shall fight in France, we shall fight on the seas and oceans, we shall fight with growing confidence and growing strength in the air, we shall defend our island, whatever the cost may be, we shall fight on the beaches, we shall fight on the landing grounds, we shall fight in the fields and in the streets, we shall fight in the hills; we shall never surrender.

As I type these words, more than 60 years after they were first spoken, they still have the power to stir emotions. I have only read the words and heard a recording of them, but they still manage to conjure up the occasion when they were first delivered. The atmosphere must have been electric – the hairs were probably standing up on people's necks. Here was a leader setting out the mission for the country in incontrovertible terms. The timbre of his voice with each carefully considered intonation exuded authority, and a whole country, perhaps a whole continent, became convinced that this was the man for the hour and that the cause they had been called to defend was at last within their grasp. He managed to pull off an astonishing oratorical achievement.

Churchill had few equals, and although men like Martin Luther King can be compared with him, there are few leaders today, unless they are well and truly hiding their lights under a bushel, who can be placed in the same oratorical league as Churchill and King.

However, beneath Churchill and King's premier league status we should be grateful for the leaders of organisations who possess the ability to communicate complex strategies so that people can understand them easily and in a way that inspires them to take action. One such person whom I had the privilege of meeting (and later working with) was the chief executive of a large public-sector organisation. He never ceased to amaze me. He was able to take a set of planning forecasts, various corporate and operational strategies and present them, usually with devastatingly simple metaphors and illustrations, to senior and middle managers in a way that guaranteed their active support for his plans. Although he had the advantage of being a naturally gifted communicator, his use of presentation skills was something that most managers could acquire, even if they would still fall far short of the genius of Churchill and truly gifted management communicators.

WORDS AS A CAMOUFLAGE

Conversely, in complete contrast to this gifted chief executive, I have met senior managers who used words skilfully as an antidote to managerial action. They were able to construct erudite speeches, presentations and reports that promised a transformation in the fortunes of the organisation, or at least their part of it. They would use the latest management-speak, which would flow from their lips and convince large swathes of the assembled audience that things were going to be different. There would be the promise of major improvements, but of course things remained the same. Their use of words alone could never guarantee success – it was empty rhetoric designed as pretence for progress. Yet their words obeyed the old dictum that it is possible to fool all of the people some of the time and some of the people all of the time.

I shall never forget the moment when I made an astonishing discovery in the area of the meaninglessness of some words. I was 22 years old, very inexperienced and working in manufacturing, and I had decided to become a personnel manager. Those were the days before the advent of human resource management and the transformation of the Institute of Personnel Management (IPM) into the far more professional Chartered Institute of Personnel and Development. Obtaining professional qualifications seemed to be a sensible way forward, and it also meant that I would escape the clutches of the education and training manager, who was convinced that I should become an accountant. A lucky escape, I think, as the life of an accountant would never have suited my personality.

My discovery took place during the IPM course's weekend away at the end of the first year. The tutor took us to a country hotel and we spent the weekend practising industrial relations negotiating skills, receiving lectures on a variety of employment-related matters, including one on the Common Market and its impact on employee rights, socialising (an important part of the course!) and studying arcane aspects of sociology. It was during one of the sociology exercises that I made my astonishing discovery.

The tutor introduced us to the concept of functionalism, a subject that I did not understand at the time – even after the tutor's explanation – and a topic that I am sure would continue to mystify me three decades later. To help the course members to understand the concept, the tutor showed us a film called *The Hill*, starring Sean Connery and other well-known British cinema stars. The film was based in a detention centre for soldiers who had contravened army regulations, and the centre's discipline was particularly draconian and administered by martinets with an obvious sadistic streak. One of the demanding punishments they administered was to make the soldiers climb the hill – a daunting prospect and a gruelling task for those so punished. There my memory of the film fades, and some film buff may even want to challenge the details I have already presented.

At the end of the film, the tutor divided us into three groups and asked us to discuss what the film had taught us about functionalism. I felt at a particular disadvantage as I considered that I did not understand the first thing about functionalism and would find it difficult to contribute to a critique of the film. The groups met and discussed the film for the best part of an hour. One or two group members made contributions the like of which I had only read in the columns of *The Guardian*.

As the time for group deliberations came to an end, the tutor asked the group to appoint a rapporteur to feed back our insights to the rest of the course. I froze, and my worst nightmare was realised – to my horror, the group appointed me as their spokesperson. Some words and phrases had been written on two sheets of flipchart paper, and they assured me that they had every confidence in my ability to represent their views. They might have, but I didn't!

We returned to the main course room and the tutor asked the first group (ours, of course!) to make their presentation. I stood up, attached my flipcharts to the stand, and for the next ten minutes or so explained the thoughts of our group. It was pure waffle combined with cliché. I did not understand the topic, so how could anyone else derive benefit from what I was saying? At the end of my contribution I was greeted with loud applause. I was astonished and embarrassed. Surely it must be applause as some form of sympathy or encouragement, I thought, and this view was confirmed in my mind when the other two rapporteurs received hardly any applause at all. Later that evening, as we 'networked' around the bar, I discovered that the applause had been genuine. Encouraged by copious amounts of wine, the group told me that my contribution had been first class and that I was obviously quite expert in this area.

Forgive the immodesty, but I already knew that I had the ability to string together a few sentences in an orderly manner, and that my considerable height, and I assume a correspondingly large diaphragm, meant that my voice resonated in a room. However, this was the first time I had discovered a frightening fact – it is possible to stand up, talk cliché and jargon-riddled bilge about a topic that mystifies you, and win the approval and support of an apparently discerning audience. An alarming fact.

WORDS GET IN THE WAY

Since then I have seen this so-called skill practised many times by a multitude of different people. One such individual was Jo Healey, who was the chief executive of a large healthcare organisation. Jo was intelligent and highly articulate, but was also able to impress an audience with a rich vein of rhetoric. When he actually knew something about the subject matter there was hardly anyone who could match the flow of language – his mellifluous voice and honeyed tones could charm the birds out of the trees. What alarmed many of his colleagues was the impressive performance he could give when he was a complete stranger to the topic area under discussion. His speech sounded good, it would always be constructed elegantly, even without benefit of time for preparation, and would be delivered with complete confidence. The only problem with Jo's contributions was that they were often just plain wrong. Yet the audience was full of admiration, and when Jo left the organisation there were many reminiscences about his oral contributions, although some of his former senior colleagues added reminiscences of another kind.

Sometimes the ability to use words as an alternative to meaningful management action can permeate the very culture of an organisation. Its consequences produce an organisation that becomes stultified in that it loses its force to move forward, and the old adage quoted at the start of this chapter, 'When all is said and done, often more is said than done', is a perfect summary of the ossification that can afflict these types of management team. Two examples illustrate this point. The first is from an organisation that recognised the onset of this 'disease', whereas the second organisation did not even know that it was suffering from the disease. Again I have changed some of the facts to protect the identity of the organisations concerned.

TWO EXAMPLES

Example 1 is taken from my work with a highly respected, large public-sector organisation made up of traditional professional staff and what they call 'general managers'. They have a distinguished track record in their field, and most neutral observers would acknowledge the success of their performance over many years. A new chief executive was appointed who wanted to improve their performance further and make it more attuned to the needs of their users. One of the concerns she identified was that the skill of the senior executive team in critically evaluating a management proposition had become a liability, whereby a forensic evaluation of the proposition and an elegant presentation of the various alternatives had become an end in itself. In other words, there were some colleagues who saw the discipline of the process, and the opportunity to demonstrate their intellectual and oral proficiency, rather than the outcome of their discussions, as the principal challenge.

As I interviewed the individual members of the senior team it became clear that other colleagues around the table shared the chief executive's concerns. One of them said to me 'We analyse, cogitate, talk up something we don't fully understand, and something emerges which has little effect on the main stream of business.' This was an exaggerated assessment of the problem, as it turned out, but it provided some confirmation that the new chief executive had identified a real problem. Another member of the team said 'Everyone has to make a speech. Our "business" around here has become words, and we've grown to admire a carefully crafted speech.' Another colleague thought that 'Everyone's too clever by half. We need to move away from "talk, talk, talk and talk" to "talk, decide, do, and review"'.

Although these views were not shared by all of the colleagues around the table, after a period of reflection supported by facilitation it became clear to all of them that, at the very least, there was a danger that one of their strengths, namely the ability to analyse, dissect and reconstruct a management argument, had, in too many instances, become a liability. Today that organisation is an even more action-focused concern in which words and management team speeches are never confused with action and real progress.

Example 2 is quite another matter. Large parts of this public-sector organisation did not appear to know that they had a problem. Not only did its managers talk in endless clichés but it was an organisation that had a hopeless fascination with just about any new fad or concept that came along. The senior managers did not necessarily implement any of the new concepts, but the phrases related to the new concepts entered their lexicon of management-speak. The clichés abounded – from evidence-based management to whole-systems thinking and client-focused practice – and the team's addiction to new initiatives had to be experienced to be appreciated fully. This public-sector organisation is not alone in its addiction, as two academics[1] found examples in other organisations:

> Sometimes managers themselves don't know what they're talking about when they use complex language, as we discovered when we asked a number of them to define some of the terms they used frequently – such as 'learning organisation', 'business process re-engineering', 'chaos theory' and 'paradigm'. In many instances the executives couldn't offer any definition at all, or if they gave one, it was woefully vague. Imagine the chilling effect such confusion might cause. It is hard enough to explain how to put a complex idea into practice when you understand the idea. It is impossible when you don't.

The organisation in Example 2 is successful at what it does, and is valued by its users, yet the tragedy is that it could be an even better outfit. Its organisational structure is such that the federation of operational groups constituting the overall organisation is given a large amount of operational autonomy. This means that local management can determine the degree to which certain initiatives are implemented, and the performance management arrangements practised by headquarters staff lack the sophistication to identify real progress in the implementation of an initiative. Far too often a carefully constructed set of words obfuscates the actual position. What is alarming is that the managers submitting the words are not being intentionally devious, and certainly are not malevolent in their intent, but rather the 'disease' of clichés and rhetoric that has infected parts of their organisation has affected their managerial response. They have become expert at describing a situation in detail, they can assess the options open to them and are content to spend many a happy hour on a project board examining the alternative courses of action available, but when it comes to the actual implementation of the most appropriate solution, they become transfixed. The complexity of their organisation means that some plausible reason can usually be given to explain the logic of inactivity. Other parts of the organisation are quite different and have successfully implemented a range of management practices. They have overcome the cultural problem that afflicts other groups in the organisation, or perhaps they were immune to it in the first place.

MANAGEMENT-SPEAK

In an attempt to highlight this difficulty I developed an entertaining learning device (based on something I had seen utilised by the inimitable Roy Lilley, the health commentator) to use with their senior managers and non-executive directors. The chart met the needs of this management team and many other teams, and is called 'How to Speak like a Management Guru' (*see* Figure 10.1). It is fun and effective.

The game starts by asking members of the 'audience' if they want to speak like management gurus. Some do, and readily volunteer, while others take more convincing. Some will never be convinced. Those who are keen to participate are asked to call out three numbers between one and nine, and they are assured that as a result of this, and with some help from my as yet undisclosed chart, they will be able to speak like management gurus. No doubt their organisation will wish to promote them immediately. The extroverts and activists in the group will shout out 3, 5, 6 or 7, 1, 4 or something similar, and as they do so I respond

1 Co-ordinated		1 Management
2 Integrated		2 Organisational
3 Specialised		3 Monitored
4 Concerted		4 Incremental
5 Synchronised		5 Resourced
6 Compatible		6 Systemised
7 Functional	1 Policy	7 Control
8 Comprehensive	2 Review	8 Flexible
9 Optional	3 Facility	9 Proportional
	4 Capability	
	5 Programme	
	6 Philosophy	
	7 Concept	
	8 Strategy	
	9 Format	

FIGURE 10.1 How to speak like a management guru

with a statement such as 'If we want to solve our quality problem we need to introduce . . .', and using one of the sets of numbers they have called out, I read from the chart, a '. . . specialised, resourced philosophy' or a '. . . functional, management capability', and before I get much further laughter breaks out and the point has been forcefully made to those present. The lesson works with any combination of numbers, although some combinations have a more realistic sound than others.

The effect is usually substantial, and it leads to constructive discussions about the use of language in the organisation and whether it is used to take the agenda forward or as a tactical instrument to present an appearance of progress. As these realities are discussed, it is encouraging to see the message hitting home, and any discussion in future management meetings that resembles three random numbers from the chart is challenged or even greeted with hoots of laughter.

One of the benefits is the use of satirical humour to drive home the point. I can guarantee that about an hour after I have made the point about cliché-ridden language, one of the delegates will say, 'I don't know what you meant by that, Stephen, but it sounded like a load of 7, 4, 9 to me'. Laughter then breaks out, and I smile and value the reinforcement of the learning that has just taken place. The humour is usually translated to future management meetings in the 'real world' when important issues are subjected to the three-number test – are we using mere rhetoric or is this for real?

THREE OTHER ADDICTIONS
Addiction I
This is highlighted in Chris Argyris's *Flawed Advice and the Management Trap*.[2] Argyris shows that managers usually operate with two frameworks – the one that they espouse and the one that they really employ. He contends that the first type of framework – the one that is espoused – is something in which managers believe so deeply that they are often willing to take risks to protect it. By contrast, the second framework is the one they actually use. It is what Argyris calls the 'theory-in-use', and it is the key to how managers act. He goes on to show that this results in inconsistencies between ideas and actions, and in particular behaviours and governing models which he and colleague Donald Schon called *Model 1*. These values are reflected in the organisation, and the most fascinating point in terms of 'action rather than words' is his finding that such behaviour, promulgated through the Model-1 person within the organisation, is often overprotective and anti-learning. Argyris provides examples of how the inherent contradictions manifest themselves in these organisations through the practice of sending out mixed messages. These managers:
- state a message that is inconsistent
- act as if it is not inconsistent
- make all of this inconsistency undiscussable
- make the undiscussability undiscussable
- again, act as if they are not doing so.

This is the best description I have seen of the common addiction whereby we say one thing and then do another. We tell the world that our people are our greatest asset and we then neglect to look after them. We announce our commitment to quality and then ignore various technical weaknesses. We become totally user-focused and then behave as if the person does not matter. We become passionate about innovation but then reduce the Research and Development budget.

Everyone has experienced this kind of behaviour, but the galling point is that there are few or perhaps no opportunities to raise the inconsistencies with the senior managers without sounding like a whinging and disruptive organisational influence. What happens instead is that employees who want to progress in the organisation hear these pronouncements and quickly learn that their careers will be enhanced if they move around the organisation uttering the same meaningless shibboleths – this shows that they belong and that they are committed to these latest innovative ideas and strategies. The fact that the ideas and strategies are not backed up by consequential everyday action is conveniently overlooked.

The people with these great (but often useless) ideas will even commission reports to examine ways in which they can implement their espoused policies, but when the reports arrive – and of course propose action contrary to the 'theory-in-use' – they are greeted with consternation and the people who commissioned the reports will adopt what Pettigrew has identified as the strategies to fend off the specialist: such as 'bottom drawer it' or classifying it as 'further investigation is required'.[3] Then they are free to continue with their merry contradictions.

Addiction 2

This is identified through the work of Pfeffer and Sutton[4] – it is the disease of smart talk. Pfeffer and Sutton show that 'smart talk is the essence of management education at leading institutions in the United States and throughout the world. Students learn how to sound smart in classroom discussions and how to write smart things in essay examinations.'

Although Pfeffer and Sutton acknowledge that it makes pedagogical sense to grade students on class participation and their knowledge of and ability to express a view on the content of texts, they also make the telling point that the actual world that these students are destined to enter, or may even already occupy, is very different. In the world of management there is a need for talk and action, yet much of the world of management education appears to have overlooked the action part of this fact. With biting sarcasm, Pfeffer and Sutton compare the world of training surgeons and the maxim of 'Hear one, see one, do one' with the practice in too much of management education and its credo of 'Hear one, talk about one, talk about one some more'. Their argument may well offer one reason that so much of organisational life is consumed by talk but typified by less emphasis on action, and that those who are able to talk a good job without necessarily delivering one are able to progress up the corporate ladder.

Addiction 3

This comes from the work of Edward de Bono.[5] Under the auspices of the Oxford Forum for Development I had the privilege of attending an invitational seminar with this world-renowned expert, where he spent a day explaining to us his work and techniques on thinking. Almost as an aside, he discussed what he called the *intellectual trap*. The trap comes in three parts. There are some people, he explained, who are so bright that they are able to argue convincingly that black is white. They tend to be competitive types who want to win arguments, and that includes beating those who disagree with them. Because of their brightness they can reach a decision faster than most people, but the decision often excludes the ideas of others (who are still thinking about the issues) and everyone knows that the most quickly produced ideas are not always the best ones. As soon as de Bono made these points I thought of a particular colleague in whose office, unless you are able to engage in speed talking and can interject at lightning speed, you are unlikely to air any views. It is exhausting – rapid machine-gun conversation with little time for reflection. If you are unable to speak quickly then you are lost and your intellect is questioned. Goodness knows how anyone with a stutter survives in that organisation. This *addiction* results in many good ideas being missed, and only one type of contribution being truly valued.

CASE STUDY 10.1: 'Where there's a will . . .'

One client commissioned me to identify examples of best practice in health and social care collaboration and to highlight the factors that had led to the success of these ventures.

As I set about my work, my mind went back to the late 1980s when I was part of a health authority management team committed to achieving such collaboration. Each quarter, and occasionally more often, senior officers of local government and executive managers plus professional heads of the health authority met to advance health and social care collaboration: whole-system thinking, seamless services, joined-up action, client/patient focused care – it was all there. And, more than 20 years later, as I examined practices in various parts of the UK I found, quite depressingly, that for many it still remained an agenda item for something yet to be achieved; encouragingly other localities had made it a reality, benefiting countless of the people they serve.

As I thought further about this disparity between intent and action, between policy and practice in some of these localities, I began to produce a list of possible reasons for such a lack of meaningful progress. These may not have been the actual reasons for the startling lack of success, but theoretically these were the only possible reasons for the major discrepancies between what they said they were going to do and what they actually achieved.

1 There never was any real intention by policy makers to achieve meaningful collaboration. It was only a series of good intentions pronounced by politicians of all parties.

2 Health and social care practice are actually like 'chalk' and 'cheese'. Although managers and practitioners have tried their best, actually they have conflicting objectives, speak different languages (without the benefit of interpretation), and mean different things even when using the same words.

3 All attempts at collaboration have been blocked by vested interests in health and social care. Those who consider themselves to be 'in the know' believe that collaboration is not a good thing, particularly for their organisations and their careers, and so they continue to kick various initiatives into the long grass.

4 The respective managers in health and social care are just too busy, and so meaningful collaboration never becomes a genuine, top priority. In fairness to them, it may be that despite the assurances of politicians the people on the ground have insufficient resources (financial and human) to turn policy into practice.

5 The people tasked with achieving collaboration are incompetent and afraid to admit that they do not know how to achieve their goals.

6 Whilst individual, local, front-line practitioners achieve health and social care collaboration it can never be institutionalised formally at the level of the organisation.

7 And finally, any combination of the first six themes.

As I set about my assignment I became aware of one fundamental difference. In the 1980s my interest had been chiefly theoretical, but now, 20 years later, baby-boomers like my contemporaries and I, with aged parents and other family concerns, understand far better how health and social care collaboration can make a real difference to a person's life; how it can mean the difference between eking out an existence and living a fuller, happier and more purposeful life.

What I discovered surprised me and I wrote about my findings in a report with the deliberately provocative title *Where there's a will . . .* I knew the paper would annoy those healthcare professionals who pontificate and prevaricate, achieving little, but would please those who get on and make things happen; fortunately my client belonged to the latter group. What I had to say would also please and encourage those policy makers who must be at the point of 'pulling their hair out' at the lack of widespread action, despite the consistent and thoughtful policy and strategic commitments produced over the years.

The approach

In true academic style, I read relevant Government policy and strategy documents; undertook a review of the literature, including a variety of specialist reports; participated in conferences featuring some of the leading lights in this area; examined almost 30 health authorities, where good practice had been suggested; and interviewed, either face-to-face or over the telephone, a sample of people. What I found was highly significant to the chapter's theme: actions speak louder than words.

Government policy was crystal clear:

> Joint working is vital to deliver public services of top quality: they must be responsive to the needs of individuals and communities . . . a public service, sharing common goals and working across functional and organisational boundaries . . . to bring together the different elements of the public service in a more integrated way – to create greater dynamism, with more efficient and effective service delivery.[6]

Expert reports commissioned by the Government were similarly explicit:

> Seamless provision is an objective that enjoys near universal support . . . We need to be resolute in breaking down barriers between health and social care . . . Organisations delivering health and social care need to operate in a whole systems way.
> . . . citizens should not have to negotiate complex pathways across organisational boundaries, these should be planned seamlessly and the citizen helped to access them effectively.[7]

The Government's policy and strategic frameworks were impressive and although the above extracts concern principles, the various documents translated these principles into proper organisational and operational commitments. A reader of the complete set of documents would be impressed by the commitment in principle and policy, the connection in strategy and systems, but inevitably would want to know whether this would be evidenced through action or absence.

The literature review produced many positive thoughts and some negative ones: books, journal articles and reports were encouraging, identifying key principles that should result in effective collaboration and/or identifying case studies of successful practice. Some of the literature, written by academics and healthcare professionals (managers and clinicians), agonised over the obstacles and the inherent and supposedly intractable issues. The more I read this type of view, the more I wondered whether they might be actually a part of the problem: whether some of these academics and practitioners represented the pontificators and prevaricators rather than those 'movers and shakers' who achieve effective collaboration.

My findings

My nagging doubts were removed when I reviewed the documents of almost 30 organisations and interviewed the sample of managers and clinicians.[8] All organisations were contacted by email, their websites were examined and key documents downloaded, some of these contacts resulted in 'phone discussions and/or interviews, and many people sent bundles of documents to illustrate their work.

The case studies and interviews revealed many examples of meaningful health and social care collaboration at the organisational level and, significantly, also distributed[9] to the level of the individual. At organisation level there were various models of integration. In some locations, integration was on the basis of joint, or clearly integrated, strategies and services; elsewhere the two organisations (local government authority and healthcare trust) had appointed the same individual to head up their respective services, thereby facilitating and significantly signalling their intention to create joined-up services; and other locations had established distinctive arrangements, in keeping with the culture of their organisations and communities. The overwhelming impression was of two organisations (and sometimes more than two when the voluntary sector and other agencies were included), co-operating in meaningful ways to meet the needs of the people they served. The achievements of many of these organisations had been recognised nationally.

One of the most surprising and satisfying findings was to discover highly effective initiatives that had been conceived and were being delivered by individuals – often by individuals who did not possess the authority that accompanies organisation hierarchical status. Time and again I was surprised and impressed by the imaginative and highly effective services that an individual could achieve. Without doubt these individuals could only succeed within sympathetic and enabling host organisations, and as healthcare entrepreneurs they set about bringing together often disparate groups of people, and occasionally individuals who might be disadvantaged, to ensure that their needs were met. Often they brought into the informal partnership arrangements unexpected participants, such as sporting authorities to help tackle obesity in young children or mental health problems in young adults, and their can-do attitude was a credit to them and made a substantial contribution to the health of the community they served and to the standing of their parent organisations.

Whilst there is often a need for an element of prescription – directing people to achieve health and social care collaboration – the evidence I discovered suggested that prescription should be more concerned with 'outcomes' and 'ends' rather than with 'processes' and 'means'. Where the environment is enabling, thus encouraging individuals and organisations to be innovative and creating imaginative responses to meet local needs, then the results can be impressive.

The various examples and the anecdotes I was told produced an apparent 'formula' for successful health and social care collaboration:

> *CONSISTENT NATIONAL POLICIES + LOCAL LIKE-MINDED PEOPLE (sharing a common language) + COMMITMENT and CONTINUITY (even during bad times) + GOOD INTER-ORGANISATIONAL ENVIRONMENT (either created or inherited) = SUCCESSFUL OUTCOMES (for patients/clients/carers)*

As I presented my so-called formula to various people they agreed wholeheartedly with its component parts. The formula might appear to be stating the blindingly obvious, but it cannot be that obvious, for if it were, more people would be applying it – including those who have spoken about the need for collaboration over many years but achieved little.

The evidence I found demonstrated that, in terms of health and social care collaboration, it was a case of '*what works, works*'. For some, that meant centrally driven strategic initiatives; for others, the arrangements were local, reflecting national policy parameters and involving various organisational arrangements; and for some, the collaboration was driven by individuals (often not senior in organisational status, but possessing status through influence and effectiveness) who were people of vision and determination, possessing first-class networking skills.

The key question

This raises a significant question: Why do some organisations and some individuals make things happen and others do not? Whilst acknowledging that there can often be legitimate reasons for such inaction, differing in various locations, experience suggests that one common and all-too-frequent reason is summed up in the oft-quoted phrase: '*When all is said and done often more is said than done*'. Legitimate reasons and obstacles to achieving progress need to be acknowledged, and suitable support provided, but where lack of progress is a result of the work of those who pontificate and prevaricate then alternative courses of action are often needed.

For the sake of those patients and clients, and their families, who need to experience the full benefits of health and social care collaboration it really is the case that actions speak louder than words.

WORDS OR ACTION: MANAGING PERFORMANCE

Many years ago I saw a Video Arts film starring John Cleese. The video, part of a trilogy of films on interviewing skills, was called 'How am I Doing?' and it examined appraisal interviewing. The other films were on selection and discipline interviewing skills. The video was based on the management techniques of three wonderful characters, all played by Cleese. There was the totally unprepared and therefore easily countered Ethelred the Unready, the tyrannical and self-opinionated Ivan the Terrible, and the timid, lily-livered William the Silent who would not address any of the real issues. With inspired scripts and entertaining acting, it is a compliment to the sheer brilliance and relevance of these productions that I can still picture them in my mind more than 20 years later.

The title of the video, 'How am I Doing?', captured the fact that in all walks of life people who are undertaking a role want to know, from their boss, how they are doing. It is natural that employees want to know 'How am I doing?' However, it is a question that is often not answered; or only answered in a way that bears little resemblance to the truth; or it is answered but not in a thorough, systematic and meaningful way. There are organisations that dodge the question or, at the very least, the question is not handled in an open and constructive way. In contrast, in organisations where performance is dealt with openly and positively, this makes a substantial contribution to the development of both the individual and the organisation.

The following real-life experiences are unfortunately all-too-familiar responses to the question 'How does your boss assess your perfaormance?'

Whenever I ask my boss how I'm doing he gets embarrassed, splutters out a 'fine, fine' or two, and tries to change the subject as quickly as he can. Sometimes he adds that if there is anything to be worried about he'll let me know.

My boss holds an annual appraisal meeting. Most of them are done in a great rush as she has other meetings to go to, and it's clear that even if she has found the paperwork from the previous year, she is having the greatest difficulty making any sense of it.

It's clear that my boss does the assessment bit because he's been told to do so by Head Office. It's part of the performance management arrangements that have been introduced and he has told us 'they are a load of bureaucratic nonsense'. If he's unhappy with our performance he'll tell us and doesn't need yet another pile of paperwork and forms to complete.

I've asked my manager for a meeting so that I can discuss with her my performance, what I see as my development needs, and what she sees me needing to do. I see such a meeting as a positive thing; she obviously does not. As yet there has been no such meeting.

We never have formal meetings to discuss performance, but I've been present, many times, when our line manager 'slags off' one of my colleagues and criticises their performance. So it's obvious performance is being reviewed, but it's not being done in an open and fair way. If my colleagues are being criticised then it's a fair bet that I am, too. I just don't know about it.

We're told that we are all professionals and that we don't need someone to tell us what to do.

Does this sound familiar? Unfortunately, the approach to managing performance exemplified by these quotes is all too common. Yet it need not be, and the following quotes represent a very different and enlightened approach to managing performance:

You know where you are with my boss. Not only do we have the annual and somewhat formal system, but we sit down every three months and talk about how the job is going, any problems, minor successes, and there is a real sense that if I need extra training that the trust will do its best to provide it.

Managing performance sounds like a challenging event, but in our department it's a very positive experience. We look at what needs to be done, how I'm doing, where there may be gaps between what should be done and what is being done, and how we can close any gaps that may exist. It's not rocket science, but it seems to work.

My manager is a great believer in coaching, and has been on a course to improve her coaching skills. It's made a difference to the way we work on a day-to-day basis. There is still the formal assessment process once a year, but every week, and sometimes it feels like every day, there is some aspect of work where a discussion can make things go smoother. It's become a part of her management style rather than an added procedure.

Management textbooks will outline the various methods of managing performance and the benefit to individuals and organisations of creating a positive climate in this area. In addition to the organisational and personal development benefits of answering the question 'How am I doing?', there is also the moral imperative. How dare we not address this issue? How dare we not tell people how senior management views their performance on the job? How dare we speak about their performance to others as a matter of gossip or self-righteous indignation, and not tell the person him- or herself? This is why many people develop anxieties about their job, why they have trouble sleeping or find it difficult to relax when they are on holiday. In most cases the worrying is unnecessary, as their performance is considered to be more than satisfactory, but they might not know this and so spend endless hours worrying about it. Some managers see this lack of feedback as a legitimate management tactic – 'keeping my people on their toes'. How pathetic! It is far better to be honest and open. If the performance is very good or excellent, this should be celebrated. If the performance is good to very good, but there are areas where it needs to be improved, this should be discussed and a plan agreed to overcome the problems. If the performance is unsatisfactory, the discussion should work out how the difficulties can be removed. If all of the discussions and attempts to improve performance fail, the ultimate sanction is available and should be used. My moral indignation about people not being told about their (good or poor) performance also applies to those who do not deal with individuals who are obviously not up to the job. Dismissal is usually the very last option, as there are opportunities for redeployment to posts where a useful contribution can be made, but there are cases where the final sanction must not be ducked.

The area of performance is one where there is often an absence of words as well as of action.

CONCLUSION

In this chapter I have emphasised the need for action rather than words, but no part of what I have written should be interpreted as my being against the use of fine-sounding oratory, complicated phrases, long words or anything else. I am not trying to turn managers into the equivalent of a tabloid newspaper writer who must obey the rule: 'no more than five words a sentence; no more than two syllables a word'. Nothing could be further from the truth. Managers should not be afraid to use carefully constructed sentences and speak a language that the best writers would be proud of, or to use words that are four or five syllables long if necessary. It is quite astonishing how many times a person from one of the traditional professions – who is steeped in complicated terms, a technical language that most clients do not understand, and even the use of phrases from an extinct language – will castigate managers for doing exactly the same. Managers are made to feel that they should speak in the vernacular and then, of course, when they do so they are looked down upon for the lack of refinement of their speech.

I am all in favour of fine speech, but my point is that language should never be used to disguise lack of initiative or a lack of managerial progress. I want managers who are action-oriented but who never become a variation of Winnie-the-Pooh and claim 'I am a Bear of Very Little Brain, and long words bother me'. Perhaps the perfect balance is to know that: 'There is a time for everything, and a season for every activity under heaven . . . a time to be silent and a time to speak.'[10]

Key actions

1 Become known as someone who can speak impressively on most occasions, as someone who is free of 'waffle', and above all as someone who gets things done – someone who 'delivers the goods'.

2 Understand what the Plain English Campaign is trying to achieve – clarity of thought and the clear expression of those thoughts are so important. Clarify rather than obfuscate, and be prepared to identify empty rhetoric for what it is, even though you will have to keep quiet when people senior to you are uttering it.

3 Deliver, deliver and deliver. That is the way to make your reputation, but also be prepared to give an articulate account of yourself and your achievements.

REFERENCES

1 Pfeffer J and Sutton RI (1994, 1999, 2000, 2001) The smart-talk trap. In: *Harvard Business Review on Organizational Learning*. Harvard Business School Press, Boston, MA.

2 Argyris C (2000) *Flawed Advice and the Management Trap*. Oxford University Press, Oxford.

3 Handy C (1999) *Understanding Organizations*. Penguin, Harmondsworth.

4 Pfeffer J and Sutton RI (1994, 1999, 2000, 2001) The smart-talk trap. In: *Harvard Business Review on Organizational Learning*. Harvard Business School Press, Boston, MA.

5 de Bono E (2003) Crafting the way forward through creative and constructive thinking. Invitational seminar held at the Oxford Forum.

6 The exact references are not included as these abridged quotes are representative of many countries.

7 These actual words are representative of a literature in various countries.

8 It is not suggested that these were a representative sample as all told of successes in collaboration and all knew of neighbouring localities that had not achieved similar success.

9 The word *distributed* is used in the context of the notion of distributed leadership.

10 Ecclesiastes, Chapter 3. In: *New International Version of the Bible*. Hodder and Stoughton, London.